PROTEIN-PACKED
AIR FRYER
Meals

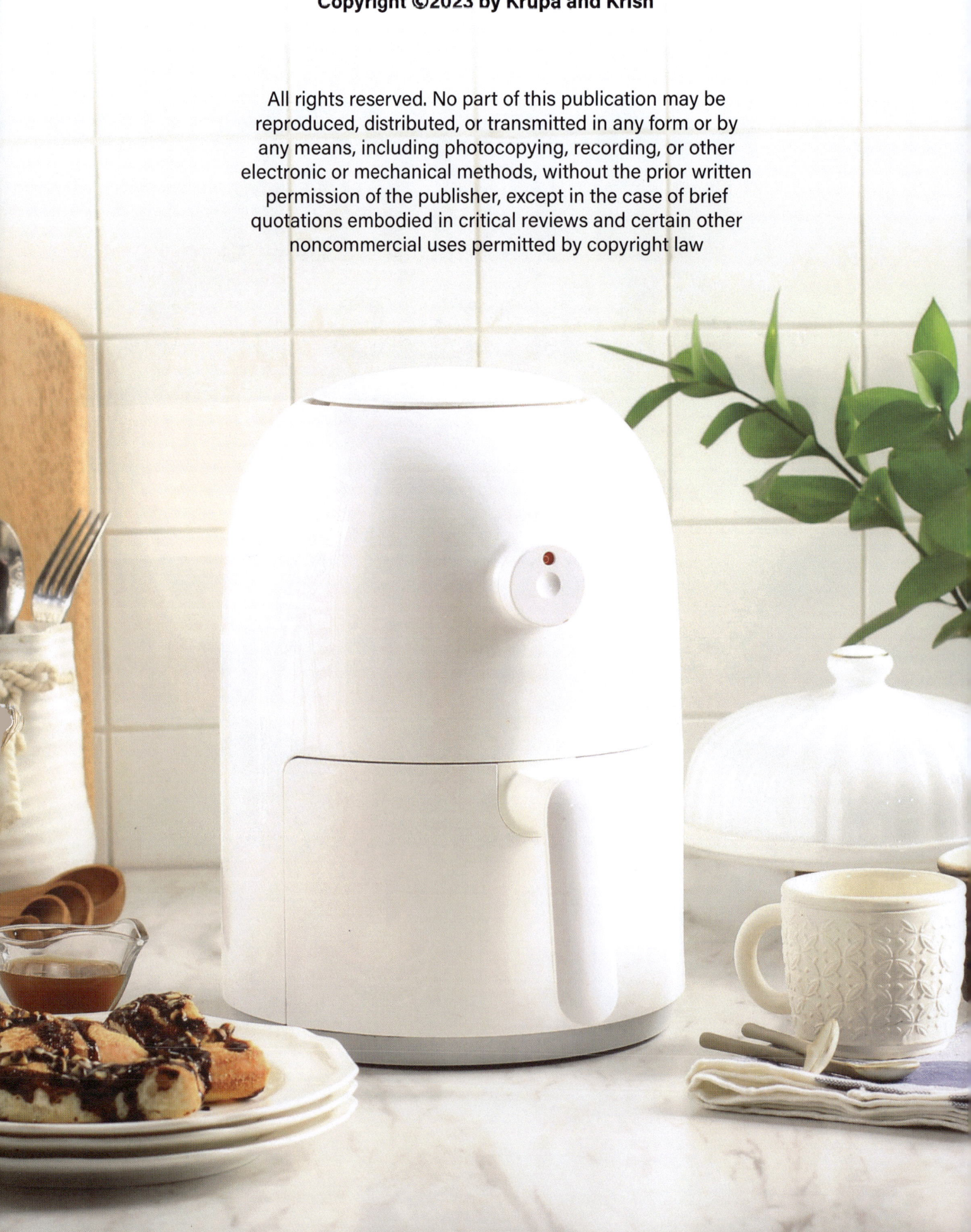

PROTEIN-PACKED
AIR FRYER
Meals

75 Quick and Easy
High-Protein Recipes

KRUPA AND KRISH

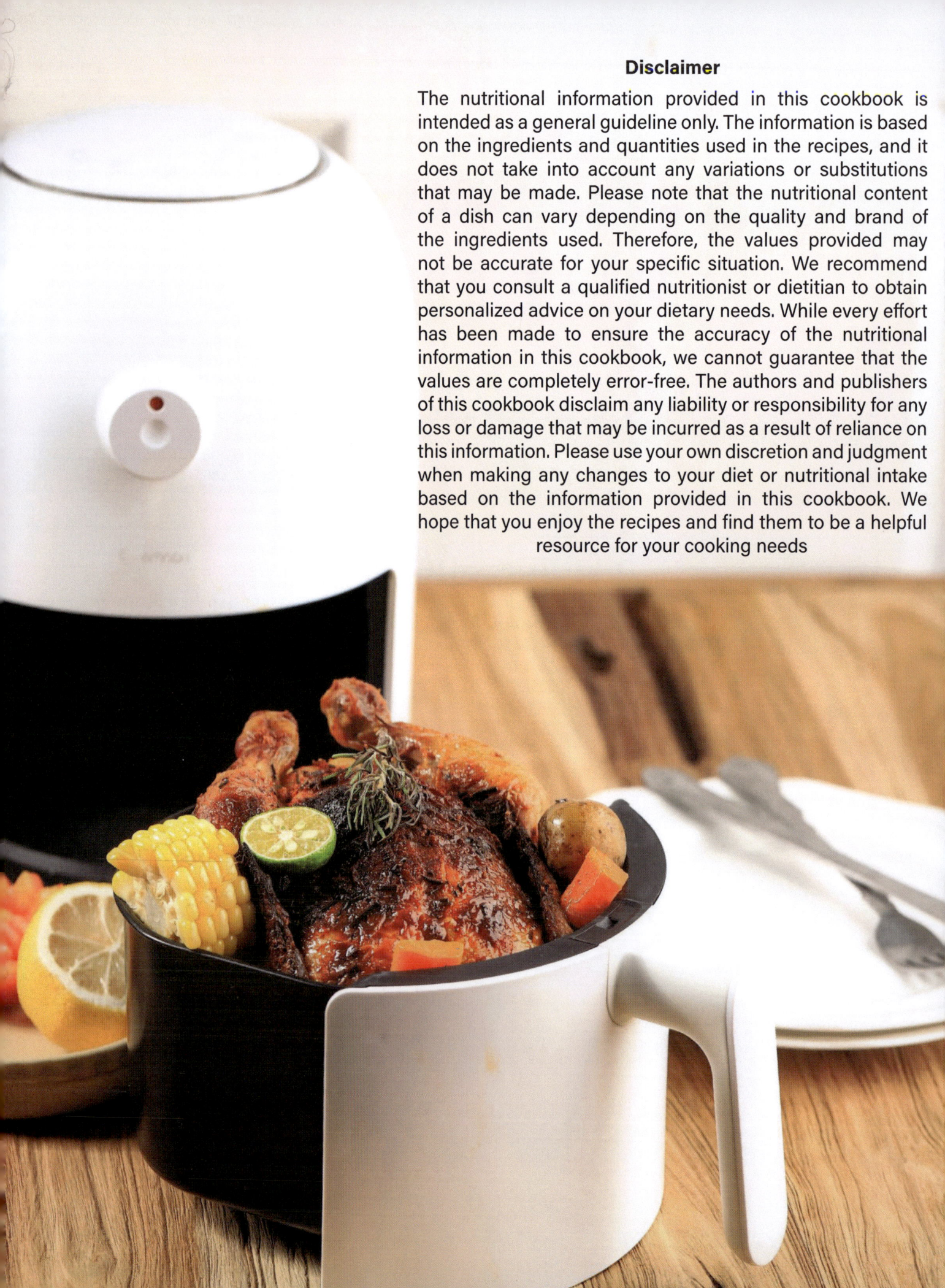

Disclaimer

The nutritional information provided in this cookbook is intended as a general guideline only. The information is based on the ingredients and quantities used in the recipes, and it does not take into account any variations or substitutions that may be made. Please note that the nutritional content of a dish can vary depending on the quality and brand of the ingredients used. Therefore, the values provided may not be accurate for your specific situation. We recommend that you consult a qualified nutritionist or dietitian to obtain personalized advice on your dietary needs. While every effort has been made to ensure the accuracy of the nutritional information in this cookbook, we cannot guarantee that the values are completely error-free. The authors and publishers of this cookbook disclaim any liability or responsibility for any loss or damage that may be incurred as a result of reliance on this information. Please use your own discretion and judgment when making any changes to your diet or nutritional intake based on the information provided in this cookbook. We hope that you enjoy the recipes and find them to be a helpful resource for your cooking needs

INTRODUCTION

Welcome to Protein-Packed Air Fryer Meals, a recipe book filled with 75 nutritious and tasty high-protein meals that can be easily prepared in an air-fryer. This cookbook is perfect for everyone, whether you're a bodybuilder, a busy professional, or just someone who appreciates good food.

Many of us in today's fast-paced world fight to find the time to make nutritious and tasty meals. Air-frying is the solution to this dilemma. Your favourite dishes can be made in just a little of the time and with a fraction of the oil needed by using this cutting-edge cooking technological advances. The nutrients and flavours of the ingredients are preserved when air-frying, making for healthier and tastier meals.

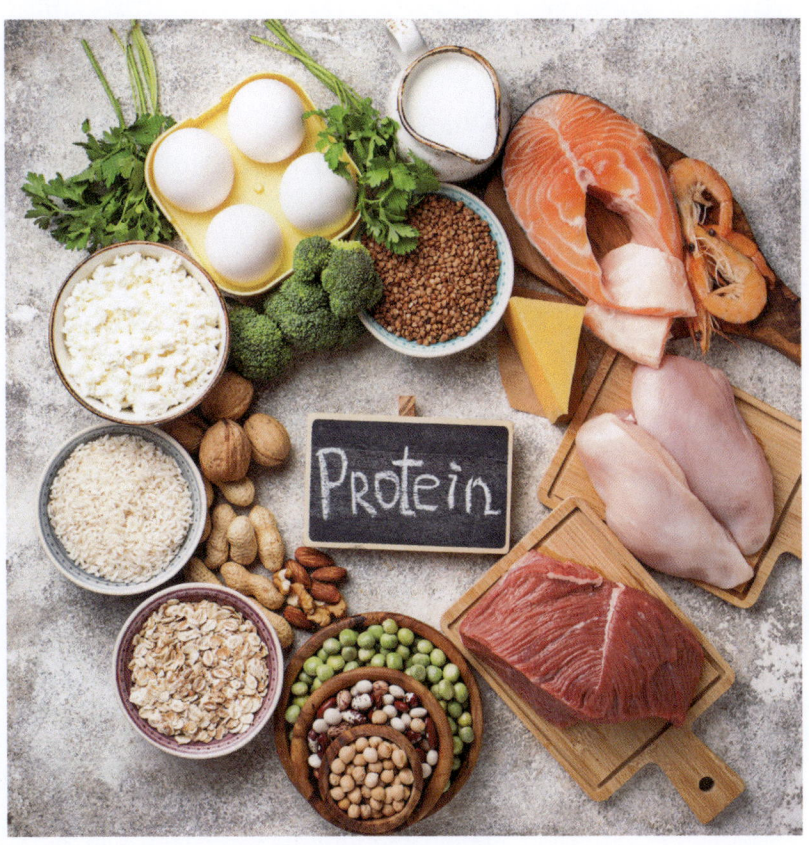

There are 75 mouthwatering meals in this book that will help you satisfy your daily protein requirements. The recipes have been divided into three categories: those with 20g of protein or more, those with 40g of protein or more, and mostly veggie sides. This means that you will find a wide variety of excellent selections, whether you're seeking for a hearty main dish or a nutritious accompaniment.

Each of the recipes in this cookbook has been vetted to ensure that even a novice cook can finish it. Each recipe includes an itemised list of ingredients, comprehensive directions, and a stunning photo of the final product. If you're like us, you're always on the lookout for new ways to incorporate healthy ingredients into your diet.

Encouraging you to explore new recipes and air-fry methods is our goal with this imaginative guidebook. You'll never have diet boredom again with these 75 healthy and delicious meals. Get out your air fryer, crank up the temperature, and get to work!

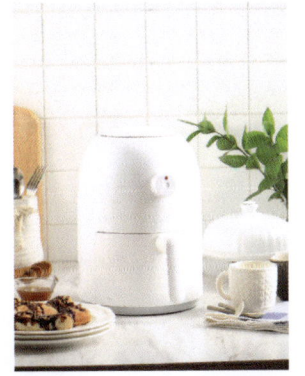
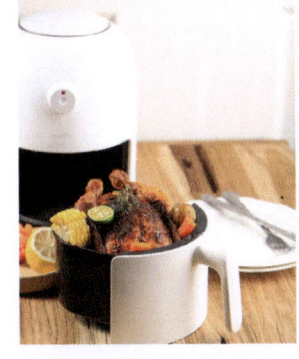

Getting to Know Your Air Fryer

If you're a beginner to air frying, you might wonder about this innovative cooking method. An air fryer is a kitchen instrument that utilizes hot air to circulate your food, creating a crispy, golden-brown exterior without excess oil. This makes it a healthier and more convenient alternative to traditional frying methods.

But the benefits of air frying go beyond just health and convenience. Here are some of the top best find reasons why you consider using an air fryer:

Healthier Cooking: As mentioned, air frying requires much less oil than traditional frying; you can enjoy your favorite foods without guilt. Plus, air frying helps reduce the amount of harmful acrylamide that can form in certain foods when cooked at high temperatures.

Versatility: Air fryers are incredibly versatile and can cook a variety of foods, from crispy fried chicken to roasted vegetables to baked desserts.

Time-Saving: Because air fryers cook food faster than traditional ovens, they can help you save time in the kitchen. Plus, many air fryers come with pre-programmed settings for popular dishes, so you don't have to guess the cooking time and temperature.

Easy to Clean: Unlike deep fryers, which can be messy and difficult to clean, air fryers are typically easy to clean and maintain. Many models come with removable trays and baskets that can be washed in the dishwasher.

General knowledge when using your air fryer.

Preheat Your Air Fryer: Just like with a traditional oven, it's important to preheat your air fryer before cooking. This will help ensure your food cooks evenly and crisps up nicely.

Use the Right Amount of Oil: While you don't need as much oil as traditional frying methods, you still need to use some oil to help your food cook and crisp up. Aim for about 1-2 tablespoons of oil per pound of food.

Don't Overcrowd the Basket: To ensure that your food cooks evenly, it's important to keep your air fryer basket manageable. Leave some room between each piece of food so that air can flow.

Shake the Basket: To help your food cook evenly on all sides, it's a good idea to shake your air fryer basket mid-through through the cooking process.

Experiment with Seasonings: One of the benefits of air frying is the ability to experiment with various seasonings and flavor combinations. Don't hesitate to try new spices and herbs to enhance the flavor and make your dishes delicious.

By following these tips and getting to know your air fryer, you'll be well on your way to creating delicious and healthy meals in no time.

TABLE OF CONTENTS

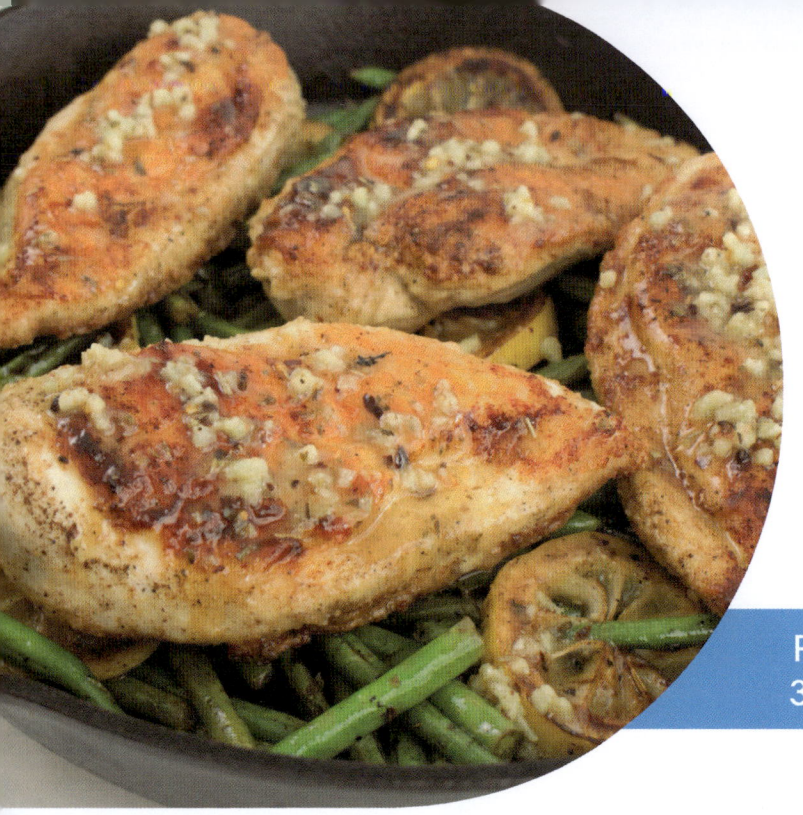

LEMON GARLIC CHICKEN

NUTRITION INFORMATION

Calories:	385 Kcal
Protein:	48 g
Carb:	19 g
Fat:	3 g

Prep Time: 30 Minutes	Servings 4

INGREDIENTS

- 1.5 lb. boneless, skinless chicken breasts
- 1/4 cup olive oil
- 1/4 cup fresh lemon juice
- 4 cloves garlic, minced
- 1 tablespoon chopped fresh parsley
- 1/2 teaspoon salt
- 1/4 teaspoon black pepper
- Lemon wedges and fresh parsley for garnish

INSTRUCTIONS

1. Mix in a small basin the olive oil, lemon juice, minced garlic, parsley, salt, and pepper in a small basin. Pour out marinade over chicken breasts in a shallow dish. Cover and chill for 30–4 hours.
2. Set up the air fryer to 360°F (180°C). Put the chicken in your air fryer basket after draining the marinade. Discard marinade.
3. Flip the chicken halfway through cooking for 20 mins or until it reaches 165°F (74°C). Serve chicken with lemon wedges and fresh parsley after air-frying.

SPICY SHRIMP AND QUINOA SKEWERS

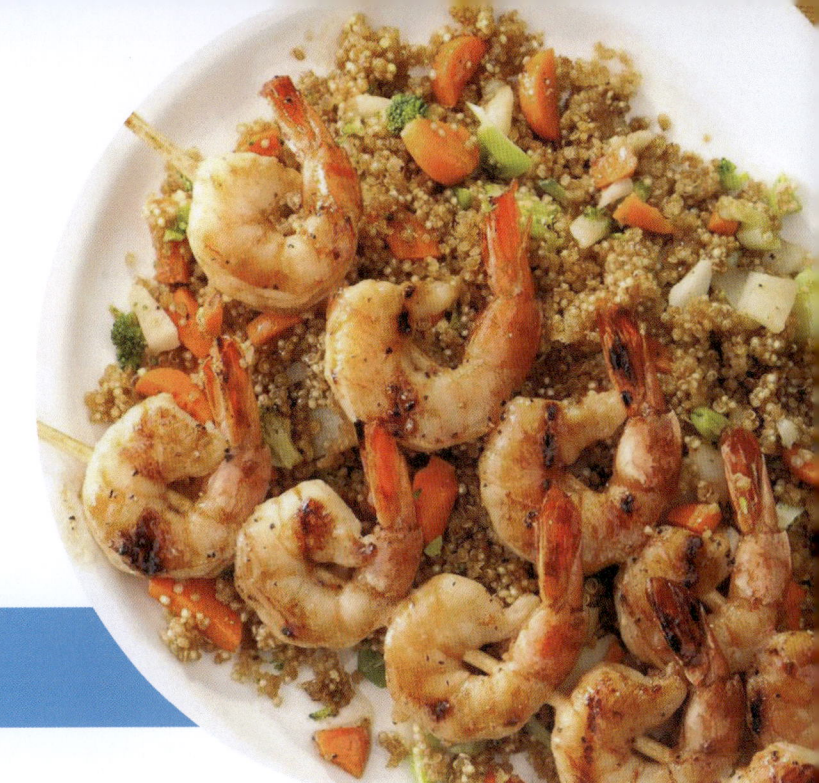

NUTRITION INFORMATION

Calories:	390 Kcal
Protein:	40 g
Carb:	16 g
Fat:	26 g

Prep Time: 40 Minutes	Servings 4

INGREDIENTS

- 1.5 lb large shrimp, peeled and deveined
- 2 cups cooked quinoa
- 1/4 cup olive oil
- 2 tablespoons hot sauce
- 1 tablespoon smoked paprika
- 1 tablespoon minced garlic
- 1/2 teaspoon salt
- 1/4 teaspoon black pepper
- 1 tablespoon chopped fresh cilantro
- 8 wooden skewers soaked in water

INSTRUCTIONS

1. Combine the olive oil, hot sauce, smoked paprika, garlic, salt, and pepper in a bowl.
2. Add the shrimp to the marinade, making sure they are evenly coated. Cover and refrigerate for 30 minutes. Set the air fryer's temperature to 400°F (200°C).
3. Thread the marinated shrimp and cooked quinoa onto the soaked wooden skewers, alternating between shrimp and quinoa.
4. Place the shrimp and quinoa skewers in the air fryer basket; please check they do not touch.
5. Cook the skewers for 8 minutes, flipping halfway through, until the shrimp are pink and cooked. Remove the skewers from the air fryer, sprinkle with fresh cilantro, and serve.

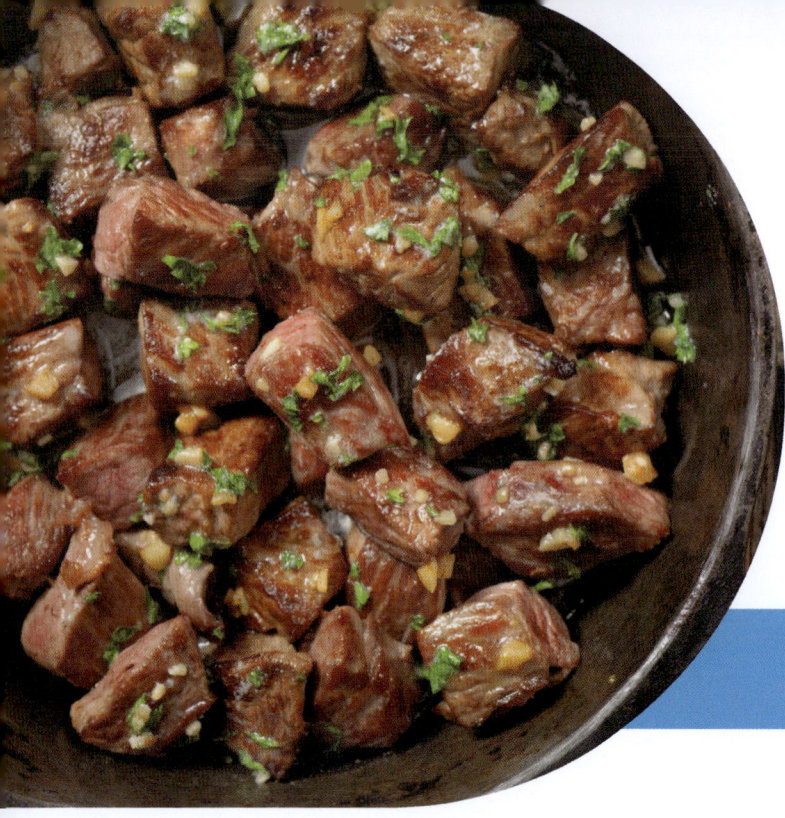

MARINATED STEAK BITES

NUTRITION INFORMATION

Calories:	450 Kcal
Protein:	42 g
Carb:	28 g
Fat:	2 g

Prep Time:	Servings
20 Minutes	4

INGREDIENTS

- 1 1/2 lb sirloin steak, cut into 1-inch cubes
- 1/4 cup soy sauce
- 2 tablespoons Worcestershire sauce
- 2 tablespoons olive oil
- 1 tablespoon minced garlic
- 1 teaspoon dried rosemary
- 1 teaspoon dried thyme
- 1/2 teaspoon salt
- 1/4 teaspoon black pepper

INSTRUCTIONS

1. Mix soy sauce, Worcestershire sauce, olive oil, minced garlic, rosemary, dried thyme, salt, and black pepper in a large bowl.
2. Add the steak cubes to the marinade, ensuring they are well-coated. Cover and freeze for at least 1 hour or up to 8 hours. Preheat the air fryer's temperature to 400°F (200°C).
3. Remove the steak cubes from the marinade, allowing excess to drip off, and put them in one layer in the air fryer basket. Make sure they do not touch.
4. Cook the steak bites for 8 minutes, flipping halfway through or until they reach the desired level of doneness. Remove the steak bites from the air fryer and serve with your choice of sides.

PESTO STUFFED CHICKEN BREAST

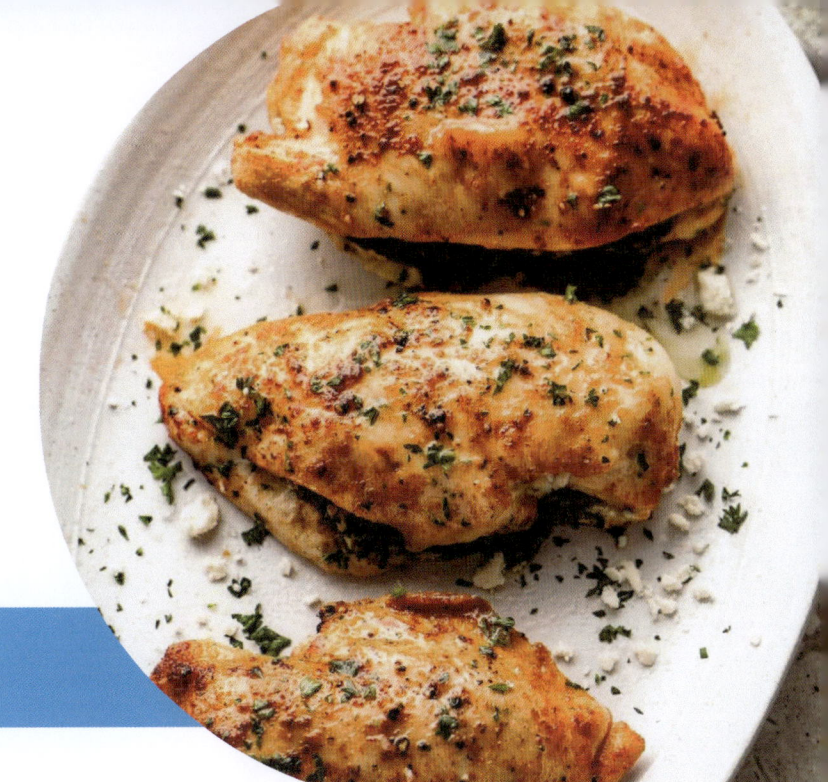

NUTRITION INFORMATION

Calories:	495 Kcal
Protein:	44 g
Carb:	25 g
Fat:	17 g

Prep Time: 40 Minutes	Servings 4

INGREDIENTS

- 1.5 lb. boneless, skinless chicken breasts
- 1/2 cup basil pesto
- 1/2 cup shredded mozzarella cheese
- 1/2 cup chopped sun-dried tomatoes
- Salt and pepper, to taste
- 1 tablespoon olive oil
- 1/2 cup panko breadcrumbs

INSTRUCTIONS

1. Butterfly chicken breasts by cutting horizontally along the longest side without cutting through.
2. Combine the pesto, mozzarella, and sun-dried tomatoes in a small basin. Salt and pepper the chicken breasts, then stuff each with a quarter of the pesto.
3. Close and secure the chicken breasts with toothpicks. Oil and breadcrumbs the chicken breasts. Warm up the air fryer to 350°F (175°C).
4. Place the packed chicken breasts in the air fryer basket without touching them and cook for 25 mins until the internal temperature reaches 165°F (74°C).
5. After 5 minutes, serve the air-fried chicken breasts.

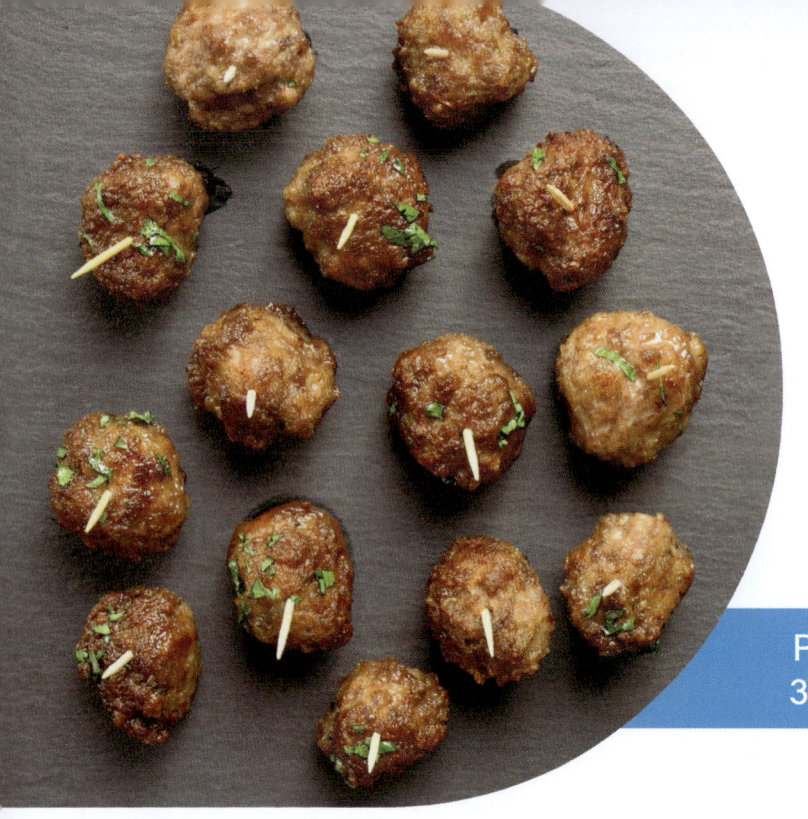

BUFFALO TURKEY MEATBALLS

NUTRITION INFORMATION

Calories:	410 Kcal
Protein:	42 g
Carb:	16 g
Fat:	18 g

Prep Time:	Servings
30 Minutes	4

INGREDIENTS

- 1 1/2 lb ground turkey (93% lean)
- 1/2 cup breadcrumbs
- 1/4 cup grated Parmesan cheese
- 1 large egg
- 1/4 cup finely chopped green onions
- 1/2 teaspoon garlic powder
- 1/2 teaspoon onion powder
- Salt and pepper, to taste
- 1/2 cup buffalo sauce

INSTRUCTIONS

1. Combine the ground turkey, breadcrumbs, Parmesan cheese, egg, green onions, garlic powder, onion powder, salt, and pepper in a large mixing bowl. Mix well.
2. Form the mixture into 16 meatballs, each about the size of a golf ball. Set the air fryer's temperature to 375°F (190°C). Set the meatballs in the air fryer basket in a single layer without touching them.
3. Cook the meatballs for 15 minutes, flipping halfway through or until fully cooked. Transfer the cooked meatballs to a bowl and toss them with buffalo sauce.
4. Serve the buffalo turkey meatballs with your sides or over a salad.

SESAME CRUSTED TOFU

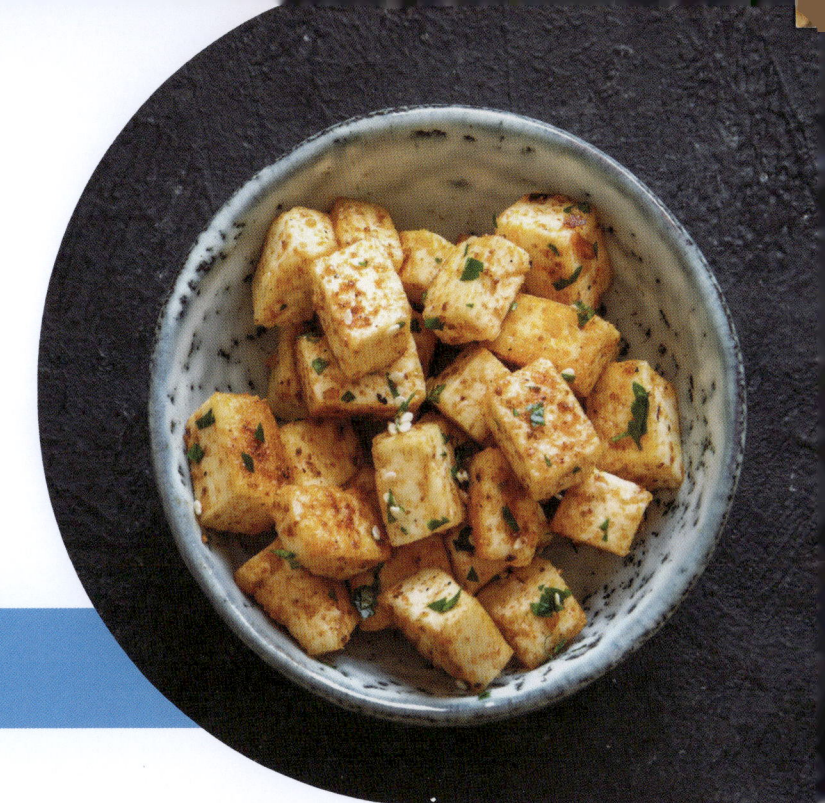

NUTRITION INFORMATION

Calories:	552 Kcal
Protein:	45 g
Carb:	30 g
Fat:	23 g

Prep Time: 60 Minutes	Servings 4

INGREDIENTS

- 1 1/2 lb extra-firm tofu, pressed and drained
- 1/4 cup low-sodium soy sauce
- 2 tablespoons rice vinegar
- 1 tablespoon sesame oil
- 1 tablespoon honey
- 1/2 teaspoon ground ginger
- 1/2 teaspoon garlic powder
- 1/2 cup sesame seeds

INSTRUCTIONS

1. Slice the pressed tofu into 1/2-inch thick slabs and cut each slab into 4 equal-sized pieces. Mix soy sauce, rice vinegar, sesame oil, honey, ground ginger, and garlic powder in a shallow bowl.
2. Coat the tofu with marinade. Cover and freezer for 30 mins, flipping the tofu halfway. Get the air fryer to a temperature of 375°F (190°C).
3. Toss the tofu with sesame seeds after draining the marinade. Place the sesame-crusted tofu pieces in the air fryer basket in a single layer without touching them.
4. Cook the tofu for 15 minutes, flipping halfway through, or until golden brown and crispy. Serve the sesame-crusted tofu with your choice of sides or over a salad.

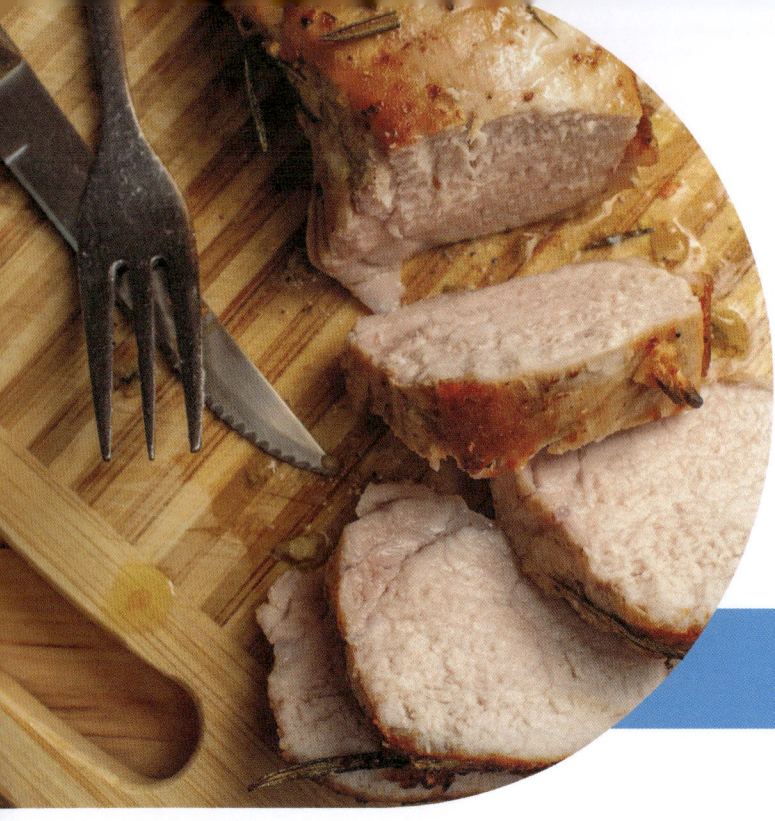

MUSTARD GLAZED PORK TENDERLOIN

NUTRITION INFORMATION

Calories:	410 Kcal
Protein:	48 g
Carb:	14 g
Fat:	12 g

Prep Time: 65 Minutes	Servings 4

INGREDIENTS

- 1 1/2 lb pork tenderloin, trimmed of excess fat
- 1/4 cup Dijon mustard
- 1/4 cup whole-grain mustard
- 2 tablespoons honey
- 1 tablespoon minced garlic
- 1 tablespoon chopped fresh rosemary
- Salt and pepper, to taste

INSTRUCTIONS

1. Combine Dijon mustard, whole-grain mustard, honey, garlic, rosemary, salt, and pepper in a small bowl.
2. Marinate the pork tenderloin in mustard for 30–2 hours in the fridge. Get the air fryer to a temperature of 375°F (190°C).
3. Cook the marinated pork tenderloin in the air fryer basket for 25 minutes until it reaches 145°F (63°C). After 5 minutes, slice and serve the pork tenderloin.

CHILI LIME SALMON

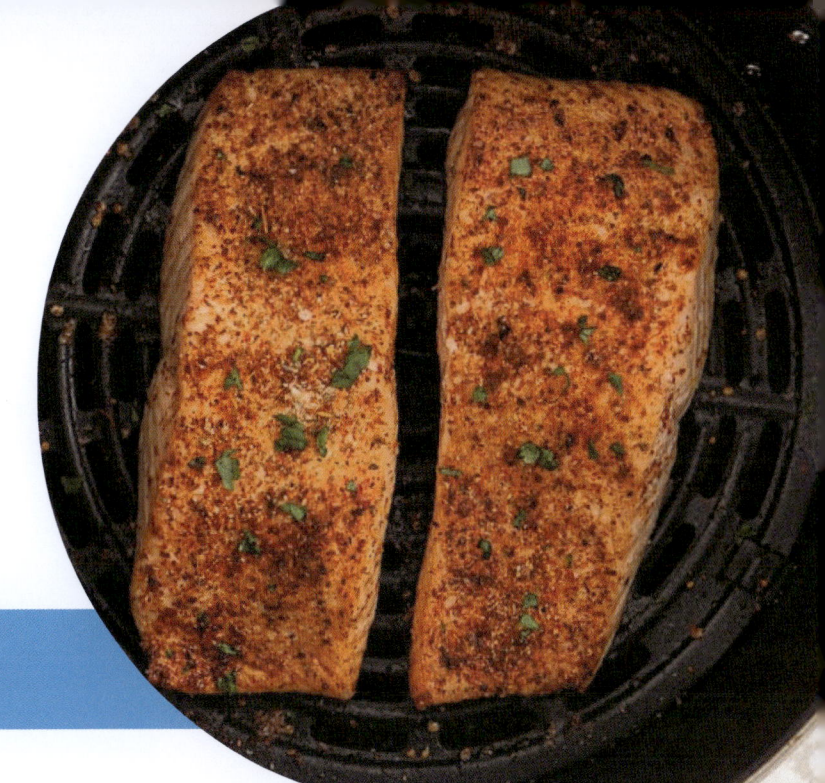

NUTRITION INFORMATION

Calories:	420 Kcal
Protein:	43 g
Carb:	6 g
Fat:	23 g

Prep Time: 25 Minutes	Servings 4

INGREDIENTS

- 4 salmon fillets (6 oz each)
- 1/4 cup fresh lime juice
- 2 tablespoons olive oil
- 1 tablespoon chili powder
- 1 teaspoon ground cumin
- 1 teaspoon smoked paprika
- 1 teaspoon garlic powder
- Salt and pepper, to taste
- Lime wedges and fresh cilantro for garnish

INSTRUCTIONS

1. Mix the lime juice, olive oil, chili powder, cumin, smoked paprika, garlic powder, salt & pepper in a mixing bowl.
2. Pour the marinade over the salmon pieces in a shallow dish. Cover and put in the fridge for 30 minutes or up to 2 hours. Turn the air fryer on and heat it to 400°F (200°C).
3. Remove the salmon from the marinade and let the extra drip off. Place the pieces skin-side down in the air fryer basket. Cook the salmon for 12 minutes or until it flakes easily with a fork.
4. Remove the salmon from the air fryer, garnish with lime wedges and fresh cilantro, and serve.

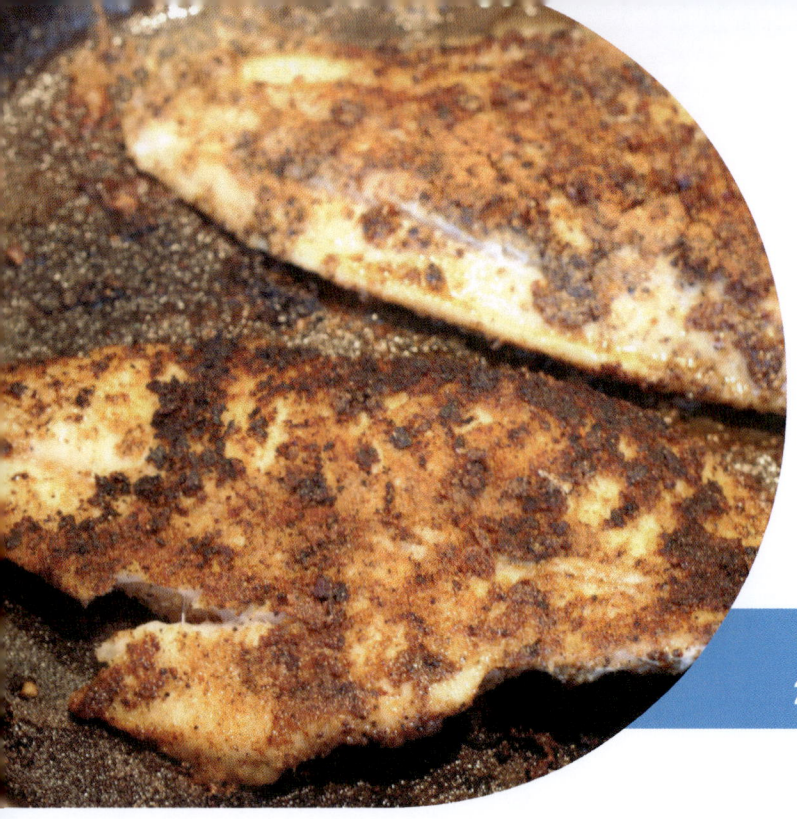

CAJUN BLACKENED CATFISH

NUTRITION INFORMATION

Calories:	320 Kcal
Protein:	40 g
Carb:	2 g
Fat:	15 g

Prep Time: 20 Minutes	Servings 4

INGREDIENTS

- 4 catfish fillets (6 oz each)
- 2 tablespoons olive oil
- 2 tablespoons Cajun seasoning
- 1/2 teaspoon garlic powder
- 1/2 teaspoon onion powder
- 1/4 teaspoon cayenne pepper (optional)
- Salt and pepper, to taste
- Lemon wedges and fresh parsley for garnish

INSTRUCTIONS

1. Brush the catfish fillets with olive oil. Mix the Cajun seasoning, garlic powder, onion powder, cayenne pepper (if using), salt, and pepper in a small bowl.
2. Apply the seasoning mixture to both sides of the tilapia evenly. Set the air fryer's temperature to 400°F (200°C). In the air fryer basket, layer the seasoned catfish fillets.
3. For 10 minutes, cook the catfish to 145°F (63°C) and a fork-flake texture. Serve the air-fried catfish with lemon wedges and parsley.

HERB CRUSTED COD

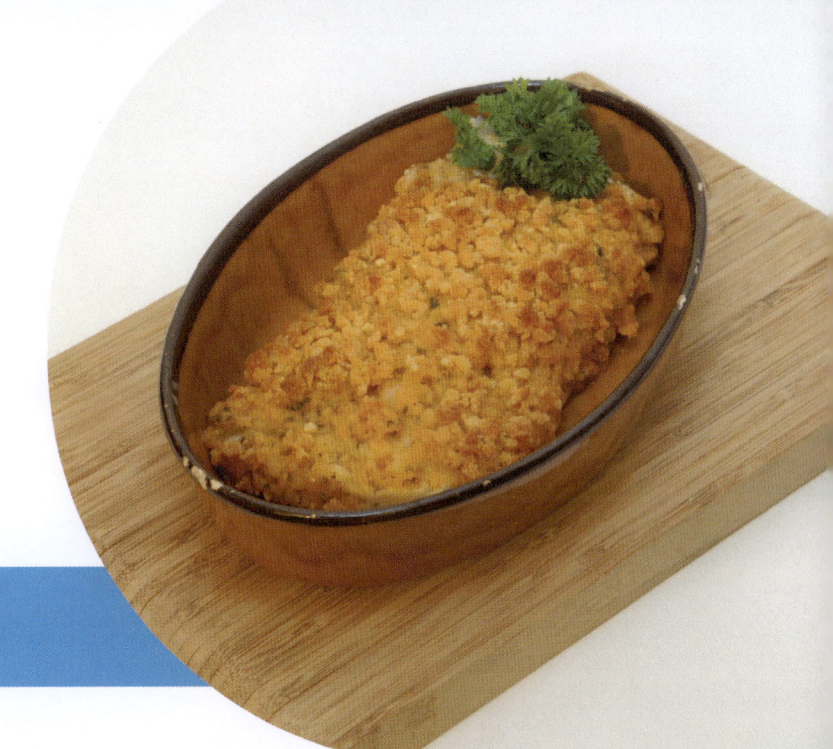

NUTRITION INFORMATION

Calories:	310 Kcal
Protein:	42 g
Carb:	9 g
Fat:	14 g

Prep Time: 22 Minutes	Servings 4

INGREDIENTS

- 4 cod fillets (6 oz each)
- 1 tablespoon olive oil
- 1/2 cup panko breadcrumbs
- 1/4 cup grated Parmesan cheese
- 1 tablespoon chopped fresh parsley
- 1 tablespoon chopped fresh basil
- 1 teaspoon garlic powder
- Salt and pepper, to taste
- Lemon wedges for garnish

INSTRUCTIONS

1. Brush the cod fillets with olive oil. Mix the panko breadcrumbs, Parmesan cheese, parsley, basil, garlic powder, salt & pepper in a shallow dish.
2. Press the cod fillets into the breadcrumb mixture, coating both sides evenly. Set your air fryer's temperature to 400°F (200°C).
3. Place the breaded cod pieces in the air fryer basket in a single layer. Make sure they don't touch each other. Cook the cod for 12 minutes or until it flakes easily with a fork. Take the cod from the air fryer and top it with lemon wedges.

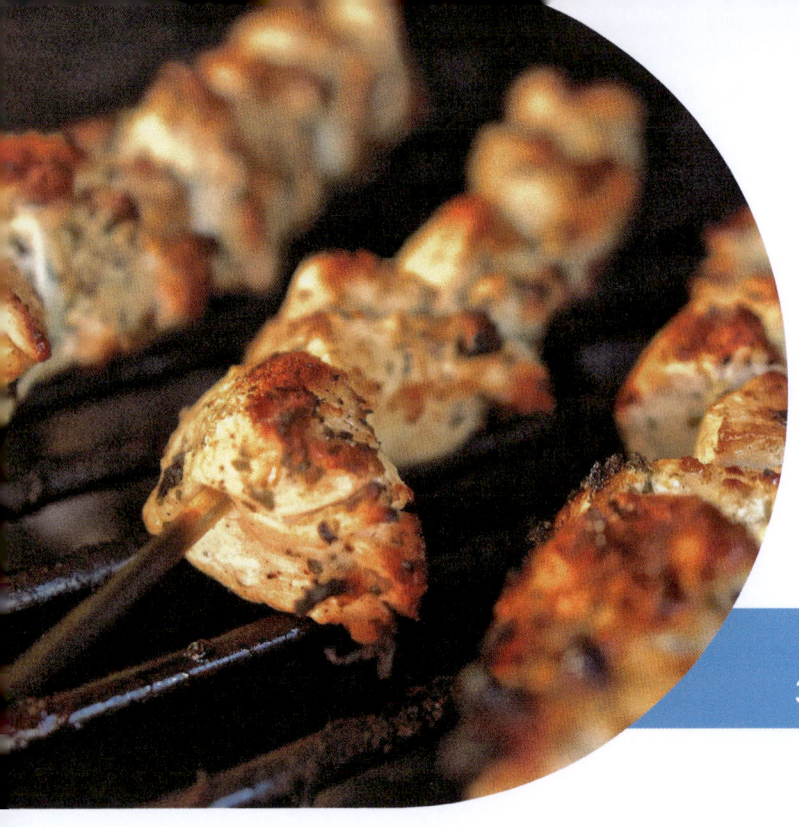

GREEK STYLE CHICKEN SOUVLAKI

NUTRITION INFORMATION

Calories:	330 Kcal
Protein:	44 g
Carb:	14 g
Fat:	3 g

Prep Time: 30 Minutes	Servings 4

INGREDIENTS

- 1 1/2 lb boneless, skinless breast of chicken cut into 1-inch cubes
- 1/4 cup olive oil
- 1/4 cup lemon juice
- 2 tablespoons red wine vinegar
- 2 cloves garlic, minced
- 1 tablespoon dried oregano
- 1/2 teaspoon dried thyme
- Salt and pepper, to taste
- 8 wooden skewers soaked in water

INSTRUCTIONS

1. Combine the olive oil, lemon juice, red wine vinegar, garlic, oregano, thyme, salt, and pepper in a large mixing bowl.
2. Add the chicken cubes to the marinade, ensuring they are well-coated. Cover and refrigerate for 1–4 hours. Set up the air fryer's temperature to 400°F (200°C).
3. Thread marinated chicken cubes onto wet wooden skewers. Place the sticks in the air fryer's basket so that they don't touch each other.
4. Cook chicken souvlaki for 12 minutes, flipping halfway, until it reaches 165°F (74°C). Serve skewers with sides or a Greek salad after air-frying.

TURKEY AND QUINOA STUFFED PEPPERS

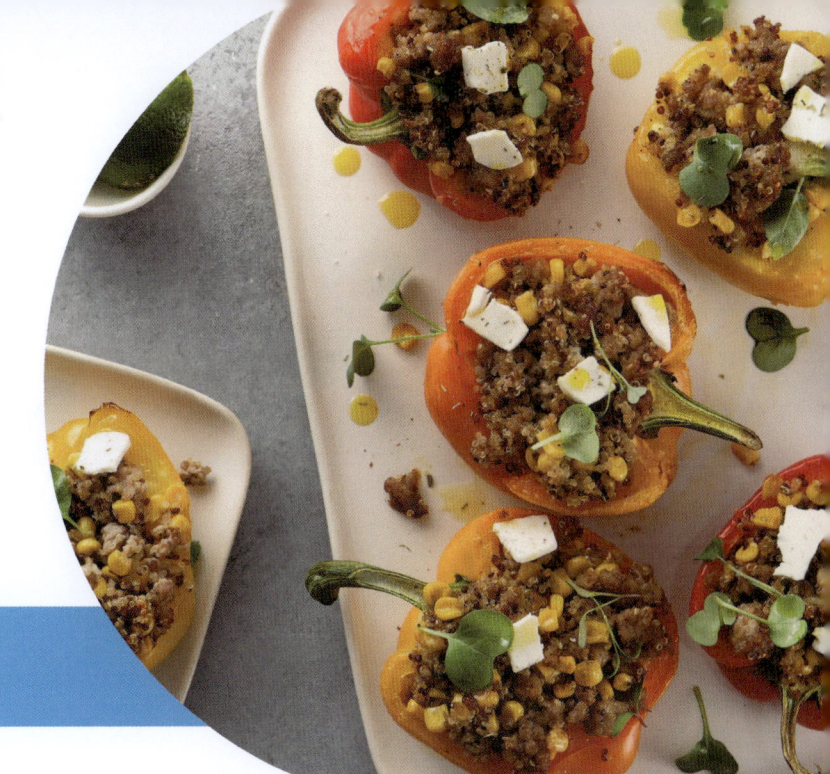

NUTRITION INFORMATION

Calories:	430 Kcal
Protein:	42 g
Carb:	31 g
Fat:	16 g

Prep Time: 40 Minutes	Servings 4

INGREDIENTS

- 4 large bell peppers, tops removed and seeded
- 1 lb ground turkey (93% lean)
- 1 cup cooked quinoa
- 1/2 cup diced onion
- 1/2 cup diced tomatoes
- 1/2 cup shredded mozzarella cheese
- 1/4 cup chopped fresh parsley
- 1 teaspoon garlic powder
- 1 teaspoon smoked paprika
- Salt and pepper, to taste
- 1/2 cup marinara sauce

INSTRUCTIONS

1. Combine the ground turkey, cooked quinoa, onion, tomatoes, mozzarella cheese, parsley, garlic powder, smoked paprika, salt, and pepper in a large mixing bowl.
2. Stuff the turkey and rice mixture into each bell pepper as tightly as possible. Set the air fryer's temperature to 350°F (175°C).
3. Put the peppers stuffed in the air fryer basket and prepare for 15 minutes. Cook each stuffed pepper for 5 minutes in marinara sauce until the turkey reaches 165°F (74°C).
4. Serve filled peppers with your favorite sides after air-frying.

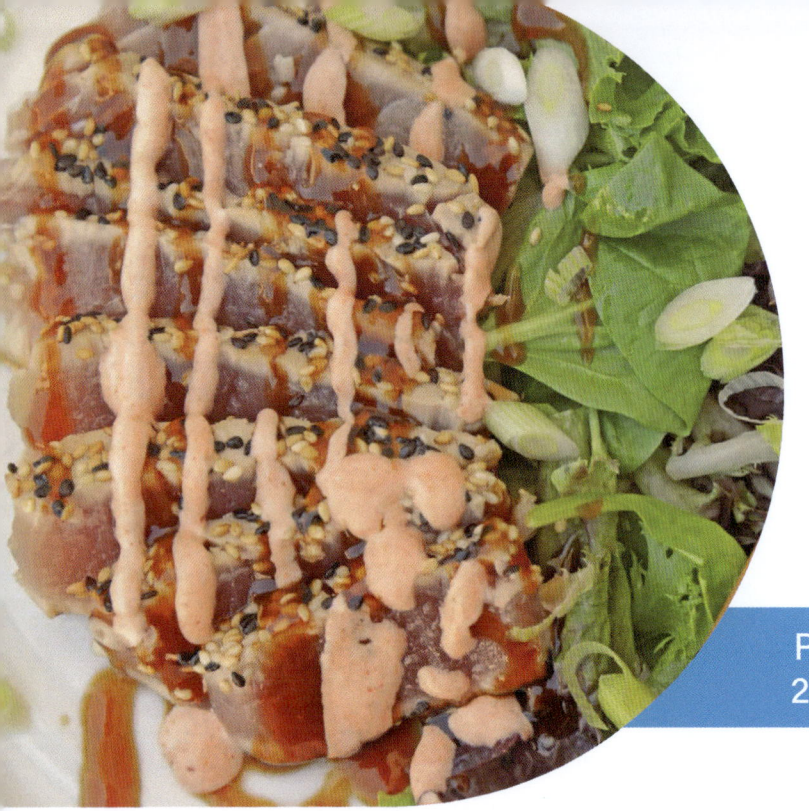

TERIYAKI GLAZED TUNA STEAKS

NUTRITION INFORMATION

Calories:	420 Kcal
Protein:	41 g
Carb:	19 g
Fat:	18 g

Prep Time: 20 Minutes	Servings 4

INGREDIENTS

- 4 tuna steaks (6 oz each)
- 1/2 cup teriyaki sauce
- 2 tablespoons olive oil
- 1 tablespoon honey
- 1 tablespoon minced garlic
- 1 tablespoon grated fresh ginger
- Salt and pepper, to taste
- Sesame seeds and sliced green onions for garnishing

INSTRUCTIONS

1. Combine the teriyaki sauce, olive oil, honey, garlic, ginger, salt, and pepper in a shallow dish. Add the tuna steaks to the marinade, ensuring they are well-coated. Cover and freeze for at least 30 mins or up to 2 hours.
2. Heat the air fryer's temperature to 400°F (200°C). Remove the tuna steaks from the marinade, allowing the excess to drip off, and place them in the air fryer basket.
3. Cook the tuna steaks for 10 minutes or until the desired doneness (rare to medium-rare is recommended).
4. Take out the tuna steaks from the air fryer, garnish with sesame seeds and sliced green onions, and serve.

MOROCCAN SPICED LAMB CHOPS

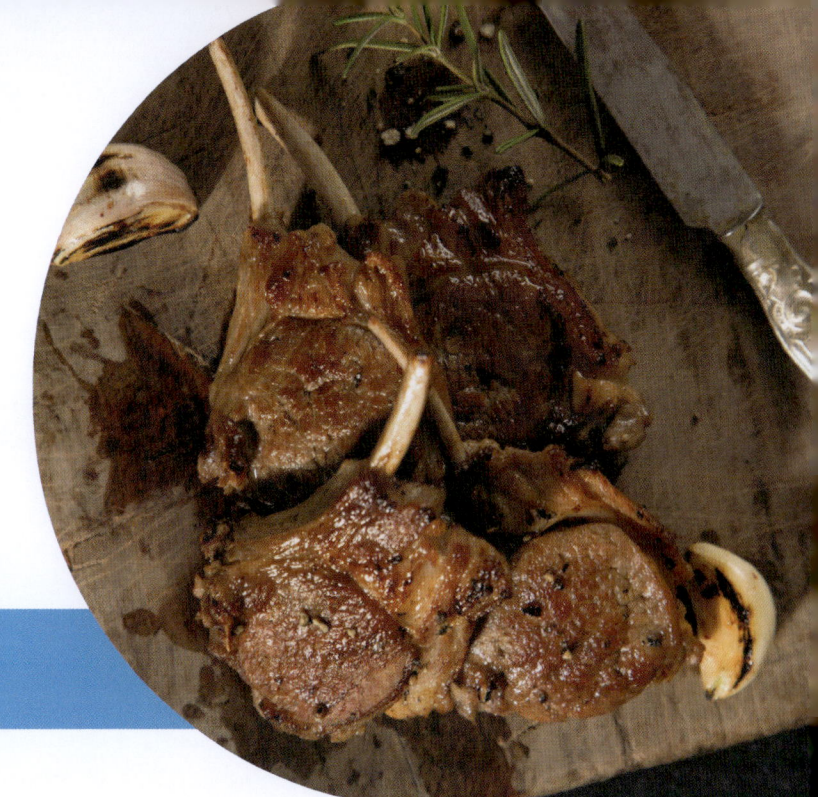

NUTRITION INFORMATION

Calories:	400 Kcal
Protein:	40 g
Carb:	5 g
Fat:	23 g

Prep Time: 20 Minutes	Servings 4

INGREDIENTS

- 8 lamb loin chops (4 oz each)
- 1/4 cup olive oil
- 2 tablespoons lemon juice
- 2 tablespoons minced garlic
- 1 tablespoon ground cumin
- 1 tablespoon ground coriander
- 1 tablespoon smoked paprika
- 1 teaspoon ground cinnamon
- Salt and pepper, to taste
- Fresh mint leaves and lime wedges for garnish

INSTRUCTIONS

1. Mix olive oil, lemon juice, garlic, cumin, coriander, smoked paprika, cinnamon, salt, and pepper in a mixing bowl.
2. After adding the lamb chops to the marinade, ensure they are completely covered in the sauce. Cover and refrigerate for 1–4 hours.
3. Set the air fryer's temperature to 400°F (200°C). Place the lamb chops in your air fryer basket after draining the marinade.
4. Turn lamb chops halfway through cooking for 10 minutes or until done. Serve lamb chops with fresh mint and lemon wedges after air-frying.

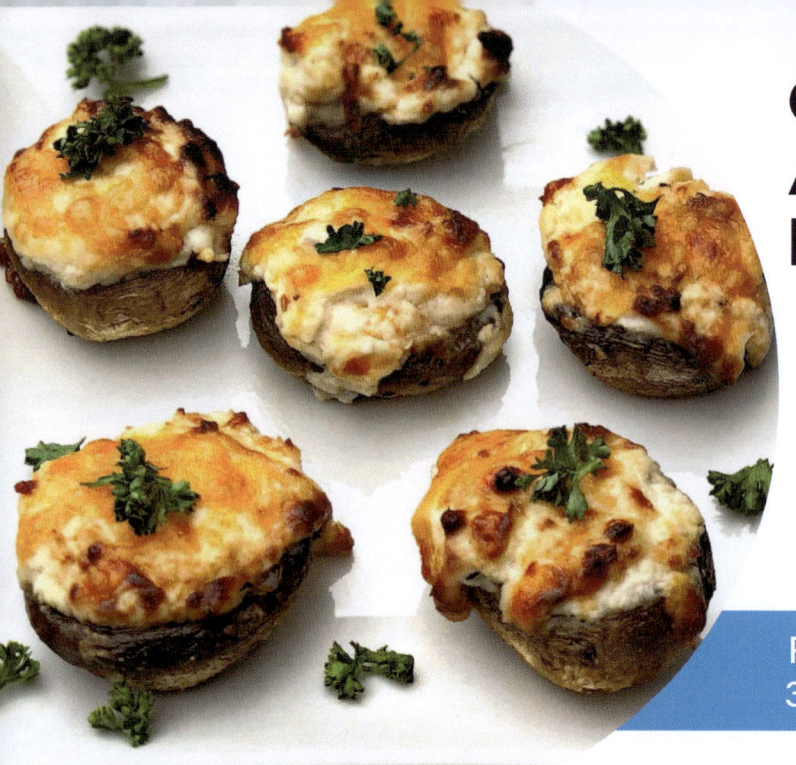

CHEESY SPINACH AND TURKEY STUFFED MUSHROOMS

NUTRITION INFORMATION

Calories:	413 Kcal
Protein:	60 g
Carb:	16 g
Fat:	12 g

Prep Time: 30 Minutes	Servings 2

INGREDIENTS

- 16 large button mushrooms, stems removed and reserved
- 1 lb ground turkey (93% lean)
- 1 cup chopped fresh spinach
- 1/2 cup diced onion
- 1/2 cup grated mozzarella cheese
- 1/4 cup grated Parmesan cheese
- 1/4 cup chopped fresh parsley
- 1 teaspoon garlic powder
- Salt and pepper, to taste
- Cooking spray

INSTRUCTIONS

1. Finely chop the reserved mushroom stems. In a large bowl, mix the ground turkey, cut mushroom stems, spinach, onion, mozzarella, Parmesan, parsley, garlic powder, salt, and pepper.
2. Pack the turkey and spinach mixture tightly into each mushroom cap. Heat the air fryer to 350°F (175°C) and lightly spray the basket.
3. To use an air fryer, arrange the stuffed mushrooms in one layer in the basket. Cook the stuffed mushrooms for 15 minutes or until the turkey is cooked to 165°F (74°C).
4. Remove the stuffed mushrooms from the air fryer and serve with your choice of sides.

HONEY BALSAMIC PORK CHOPS

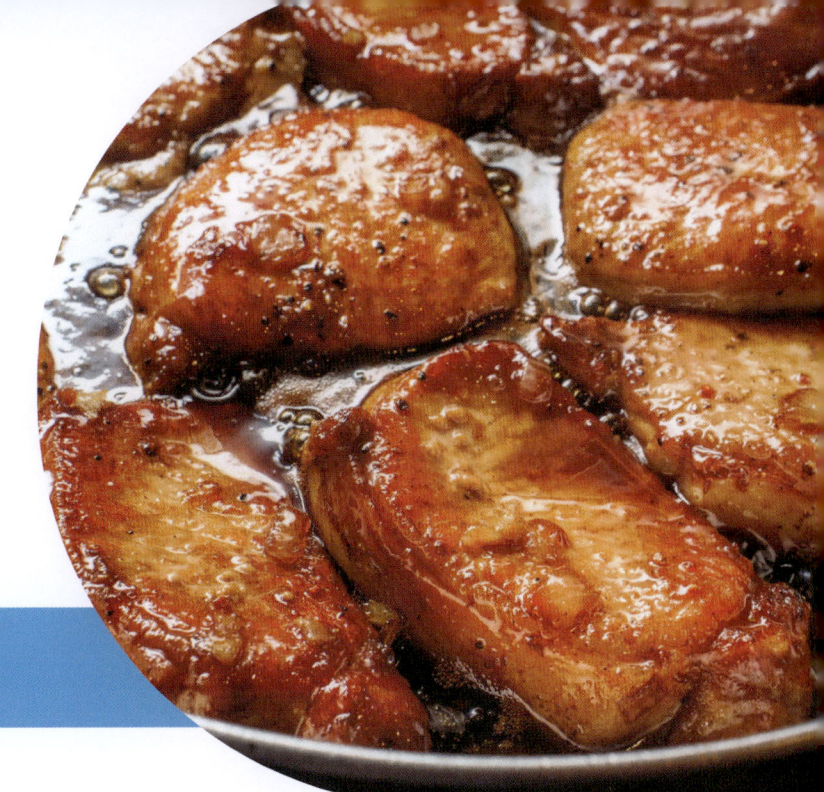

NUTRITION INFORMATION

Calories:	410 Kcal
Protein:	40 g
Carb:	24 g
Fat:	18 g

Prep Time: 22 Minutes	Servings 4

INGREDIENTS

- 4 boneless pork chops (6 oz each)
- 1/4 cup balsamic vinegar
- 1/4 cup honey
- 2 tablespoons olive oil
- 2 tablespoons soy sauce
- 2 cloves garlic, minced
- Salt and pepper, to taste

INSTRUCTIONS

1. Mix balsamic vinegar, honey, olive oil, soy sauce, garlic, salt, and pepper in a shallow bowl.
2. Coat pork chops in the marinade. Cover and refrigerate for 30–2 hours. Turn the air fryer on and heat it to 400°F (200°C).
3. Set the pork chops in the air fryer basket after draining the marinade. Turn the pork chops halfway through and cook for 12 minutes to 145°F (63°C). Serve the pork chops with your favorite sides after air-frying.

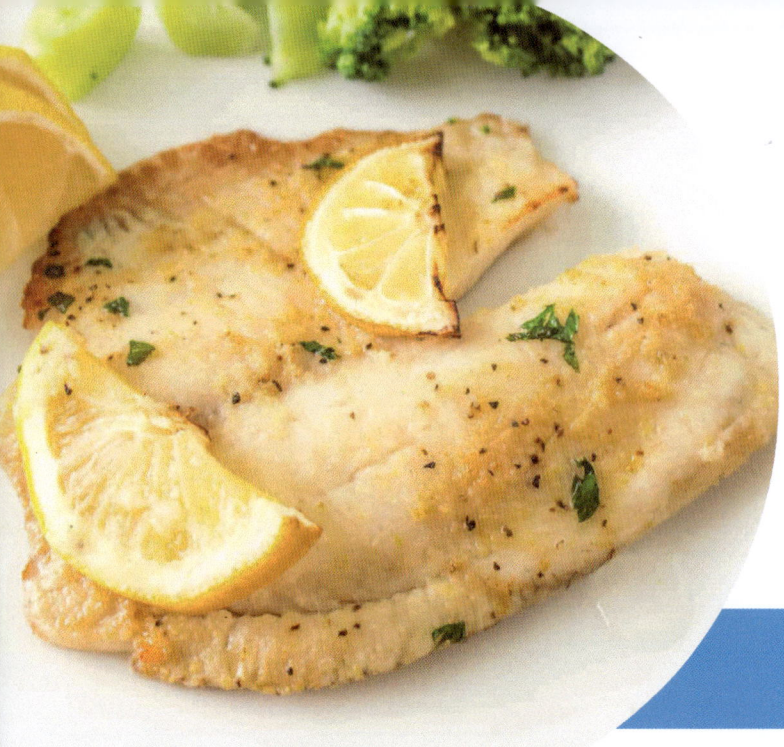

LEMON PEPPER TILAPIA

NUTRITION INFORMATION

Calories:	355 Kcal
Protein:	26 g
Carb:	0 g
Fat:	3.5 g

Prep Time: 15 Minutes	Servings 4

INGREDIENTS

- 4 tilapia fillets (6 oz each)
- 2 tablespoons olive oil
- 1 tablespoon lemon juice
- 1 tablespoon lemon pepper seasoning
- Salt, to taste

INSTRUCTIONS

1. Combine the olive oil, lemon juice, lemon pepper seasoning, and salt in a shallow dish. Add the tilapia fillets to the marinade, ensuring they are well-coated. Heat the air fryer's temperature to 400°F (200°C).
2. Put one layer of tilapia pieces in the basket of the air fryer. Cook the tilapia for 10 minutes or until the fish flakes easily with a fork. Remove the tilapia from the air fryer and serve with your choice of sides.

ITALIAN SAUSAGE AND PEPPERS

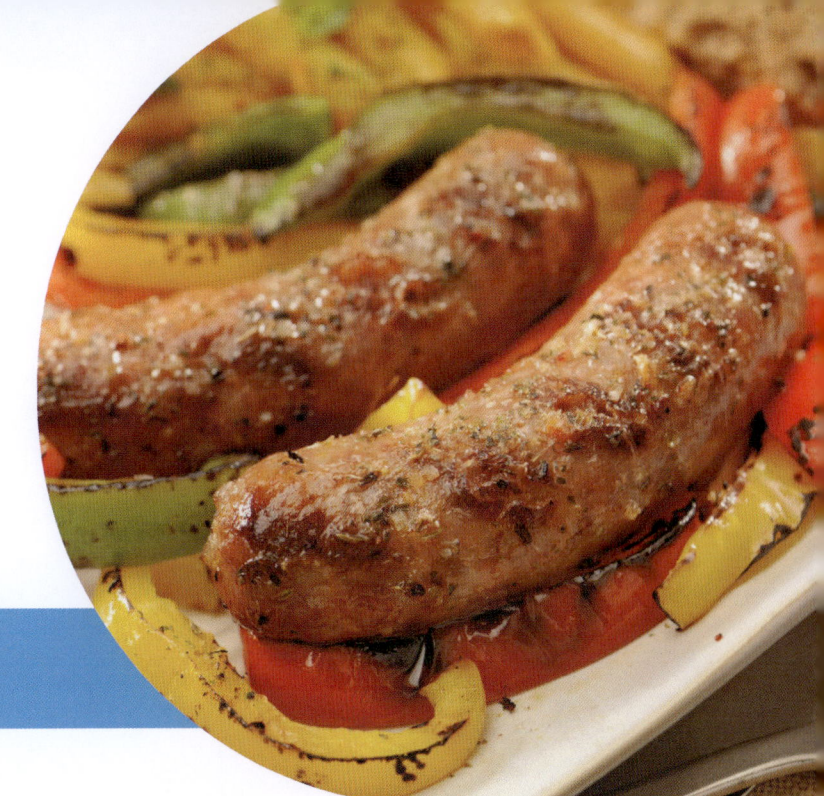

NUTRITION INFORMATION

Calories:	410 Kcal
Protein:	42 g
Carb:	9 g
Fat:	22 g

Prep Time: 25 Minutes	Servings 4

INGREDIENTS

- 1 lb Italian sausage links
- 2 bell peppers, sliced
- 1 large onion, sliced
- 1 tablespoon olive oil
- Salt and pepper, to taste

INSTRUCTIONS

1. Combine the sliced bell peppers, onion, olive oil, salt, and pepper in a large bowl. Toss to coat the vegetables evenly.
2. Set the air fryer's temperature to 380°F (193°C). Place the Italian sausage links and the seasoned vegetables in the air fryer basket, ensuring they do not touch.
3. Cook for 15 mins, shaking the basket halfway through, or until the sausage reaches an internal temperature of 160°F (71°C) and the vegetables are tender. Remove the sausage and peppers from the air fryer and serve with your choice of sides.

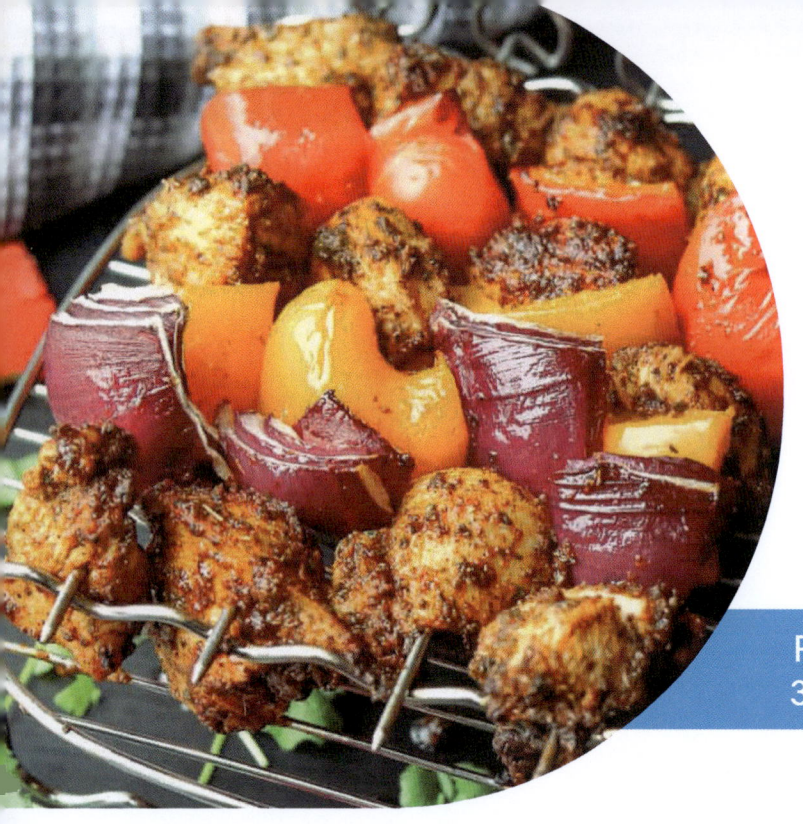

CHICKEN FAJITA KEBABS

NUTRITION INFORMATION

Calories:	310 Kcal
Protein:	40 g
Carb:	11 g
Fat:	18 g

Prep Time: 30 Minutes	Servings 4

INGREDIENTS

- 1.5 lb boneless, skinless breasts of chicken cut into 1-inch cubes
- 1 large bell pepper, cut into pieces
- 1 large onion, cut into 1-inch pieces
- 1/4 cup olive oil
- 1/4 cup lime juice
- 1 tablespoon chili powder
- 1 teaspoon cumin
- 1 teaspoon paprika
- Salt and pepper, to taste
- 8 wooden skewers soaked in water

INSTRUCTIONS

1. Combine the olive oil, lime juice, chili powder, cumin, paprika, salt, and pepper in a shallow dish.
2. Add the chicken cubes to the marinade, ensuring they are well-coated. Refrigerate for at least 30 mins and up to 2 hours, covered. Set up the air fryer to 400°F (200°C).
3. Alternately thread marinated chicken, bell pepper, and onion onto moistened wooden skewers.
4. Single-layer the skewers in the air fryer basket. Cook the skewers for 10 minutes, flipping halfway, until the chicken is cooked to 165°F (74°C).
5. Remove the chicken fajita kebabs from the air fryer and serve with your choice of sides.

SRIRACHA GLAZED HALIBUT

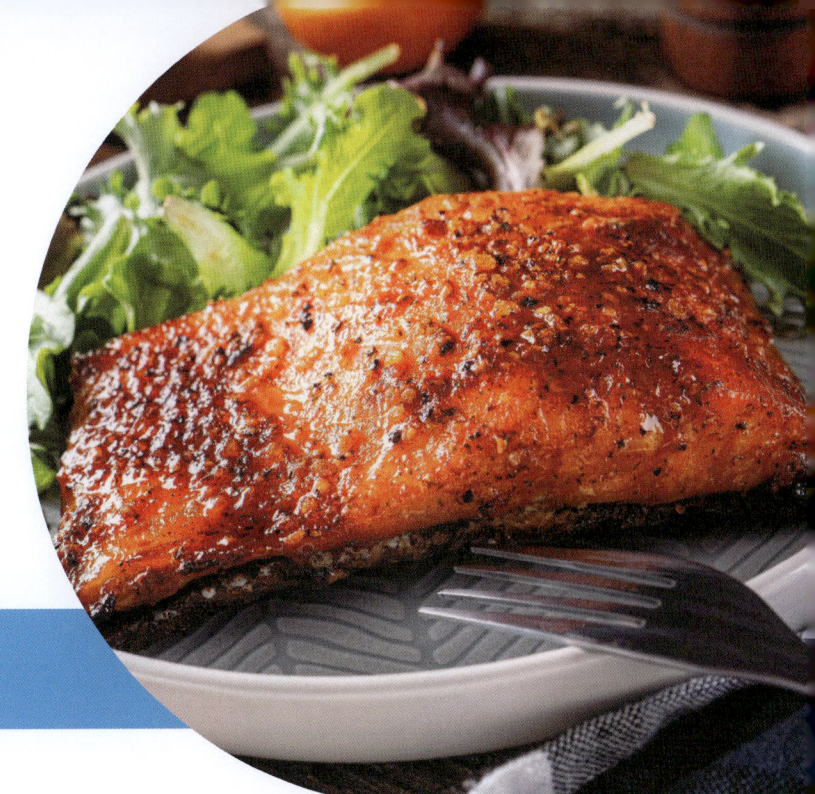

NUTRITION INFORMATION

Calories:	330 Kcal
Protein:	41 g
Carb:	28 g
Fat:	5 g

Prep Time: 20 Minutes	Servings 4

INGREDIENTS

- 4 halibut fillets (6 oz each)
- 1/4 cup sriracha sauce
- 1/4 cup honey
- 2 tablespoons soy sauce
- 1 tablespoon minced garlic
- 1 tablespoon grated fresh ginger

INSTRUCTIONS

1. Combine the sriracha sauce, honey, soy sauce, minced garlic, and grated ginger in a shallow dish. Add the halibut fillets to the marinade, ensuring they are well-coated. Freeze for at least 30 mins and up to 2 hours, covered.
2. Set the air fryer's temperature to 400°F (200°C). After draining the marinade, arrange the halibut fillets in your air fryer in one layer.
3. Halibut should reach 145°F (63°C) and flake readily after 10 minutes.
4. Serve halibut with your favorite sides after air-frying.

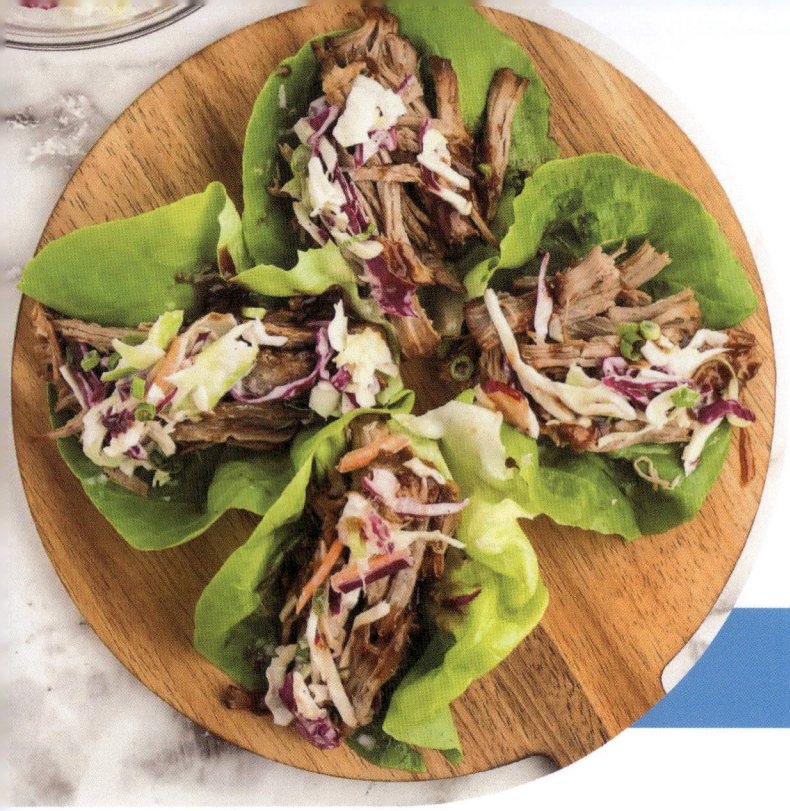

BBQ PULLED PORK LETTUCE WRAPS

NUTRITION INFORMATION

Calories:	340 Kcal
Protein:	40 g
Carb:	30 g
Fat:	6 g

Prep Time: 30 Minutes	Servings 4

INGREDIENTS

- 1 lb of boneless pork loin, cut into 1-inch cubes
- 1 cup barbecue sauce
- 1/4 cup water
- 1 tablespoon apple cider vinegar
- 1/2 teaspoon smoked paprika
- 1/2 teaspoon garlic powder
- Salt and pepper, to taste
- 8 large lettuce leaves

INSTRUCTIONS

1. Mix barbecue sauce, water, apple cider vinegar, smoked paprika, garlic powder, salt & pepper in a large bowl.
2. Add the pork cubes to the sauce mixture and marinate them thoroughly.
3. Set up the air fryer to 375°F (190°C). Single-layer the sauced pork cubes in the air fryer basket.
4. Shake the basket midway through cooking the pork for 20 minutes until it reaches 145°F (63°C).
5. Cut the pork with two forks after removing it from the air fryer. Spoon the shredded pork onto the lettuce leaves and serve with your choice of toppings.

MEDITERRANEAN STUFFED CHICKEN

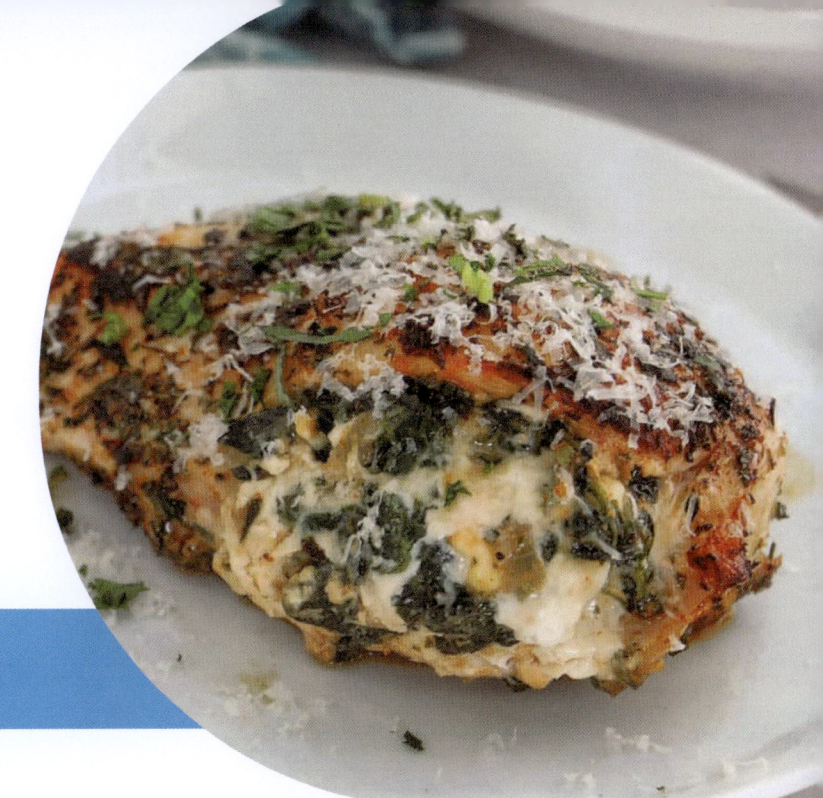

NUTRITION INFORMATION

Calories:	420 Kcal
Protein:	43 g
Carb:	13 g
Fat:	18 g

Prep Time: 40 Minutes	Servings 4

INGREDIENTS

- 1.5 lb. boneless, skinless breasts of chicken (6 oz. each)
- 4 oz crumbled feta cheese
- 1/4 cup chopped sun-dried tomatoes
- 1/4 cup chopped kalamata olives
- 1/4 cup chopped fresh basil
- 1 tablespoon olive oil
- Salt and pepper, to taste

INSTRUCTIONS

1. Cut a horizontal slit into the thickest part of each chicken breast, creating a pocket for the filling. Combine the feta cheese, sun-dried tomatoes, kalamata olives, and basil in a small mixing bowl.
2. Stuff each chicken breast pocket with an equal amount of the feta mixture. Season salt and pepper on the outside of the chicken breasts and rub them with olive oil.
3. Set the air fryer's temperature to 375°F (190°C). Place packed chicken breasts in the air fryer basket without touching them.
4. The chicken should achieve 165 degrees Fahrenheit (74 degrees Celsius) after 25 minutes. Remove the air-fried chicken breasts with filling and serve with your preferred side dish.

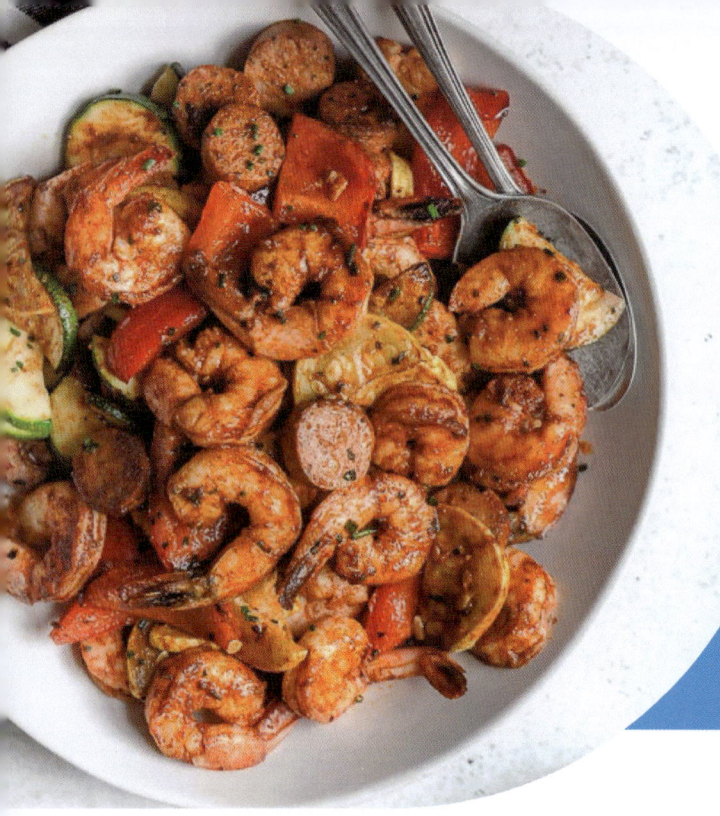

CAJUN SHRIMP AND SAUSAGE

NUTRITION INFORMATION

Calories:	400 Kcal
Protein:	40 g
Carb:	6 g
Fat:	22 g

Prep Time: 20 Minutes	Servings 4

INGREDIENTS

- 1.5 lb large shrimp, peeled and deveined
- 12 oz andouille sausage, sliced into 1/2-inch rounds
- 2 tablespoons olive oil
- 2 tablespoons Cajun seasoning
- 1/4 teaspoon cayenne pepper (optional)
- Salt and pepper, to taste

INSTRUCTIONS

1. In a large mixing bowl, combine the shrimp, sausage, olive oil, Cajun seasoning, cayenne pepper (if using), salt, and pepper. Toss to coat the shrimp and sausage evenly.
2. Warm up the air fryer to 400°F (200°C). Place the shrimp and sausage in one layer in your air fryer basket, ensuring they do not come into contact.
3. Cook the shrimp for 10 minutes, shaking the basket midway through, until pink and cooked. Remove the Cajun shrimp and sausage from the air fryer and serve with your sides.

CHICKEN SATAY WITH PEANUT SAUCE

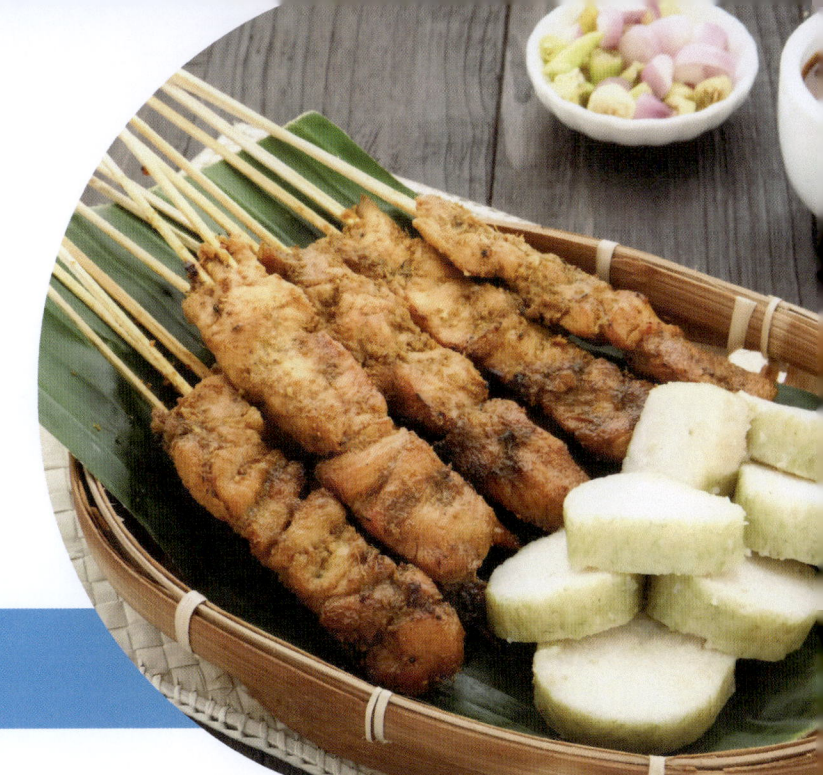

NUTRITION INFORMATION

Calories:	400 Kcal
Protein:	40 g
Carb:	19 g
Fat:	22 g

Prep Time: 30 Minutes	Servings 4

INGREDIENTS

- 1.5 lb boneless, skinless breasts of chicken cut into 1-inch strips
- 1/4 cup coconut milk
- 2 tablespoons soy sauce
- 2 tablespoons lime juice
- 1 tablespoon brown sugar
- 1 tablespoon grated fresh ginger
- 1 tablespoon curry powder
- Salt and pepper, to taste
- 8 wooden skewers soaked in water

Peanut Sauce
- 1/2 cup smooth peanut
- 1/4 cup coconut milk
- 2 tablespoons lime juice
- 2 tablespoons soy sauce
- 1 tablespoon brown sugar
- 1 tablespoon grated fresh ginger
- 1 clove garlic, minced
- 1/4 tsp crushed red pepper flakes (optional)

INSTRUCTIONS

1. Combine the coconut milk, soy sauce, lime juice, brown sugar, ginger, curry powder, salt, and pepper in a shallow dish.
2. Add the chicken strips to the marinade, ensuring they are well-coated. Cover and put in the fridge for 30 minutes or up to 2 hours. Turn the air fryer on and heat it to 400°F (200°C).
3. Thread marinated chicken strips onto moistened wooden skewers. Put one layer of skewers in the basket of the air fryer.
4. Cook the skewers for 10 minutes, flipping halfway, until the chicken is cooked to 165°F (74°C).

Peanut Sauce:

5. Mix peanut butter, coconut milk, lime juice, soy sauce, brown sugar, ginger, garlic, and crushed red pepper flakes in a bowl. Stir until the mixture is smooth.
6. Remove the chicken satay skewers from the air fryer and serve with the peanut sauce for dipping.

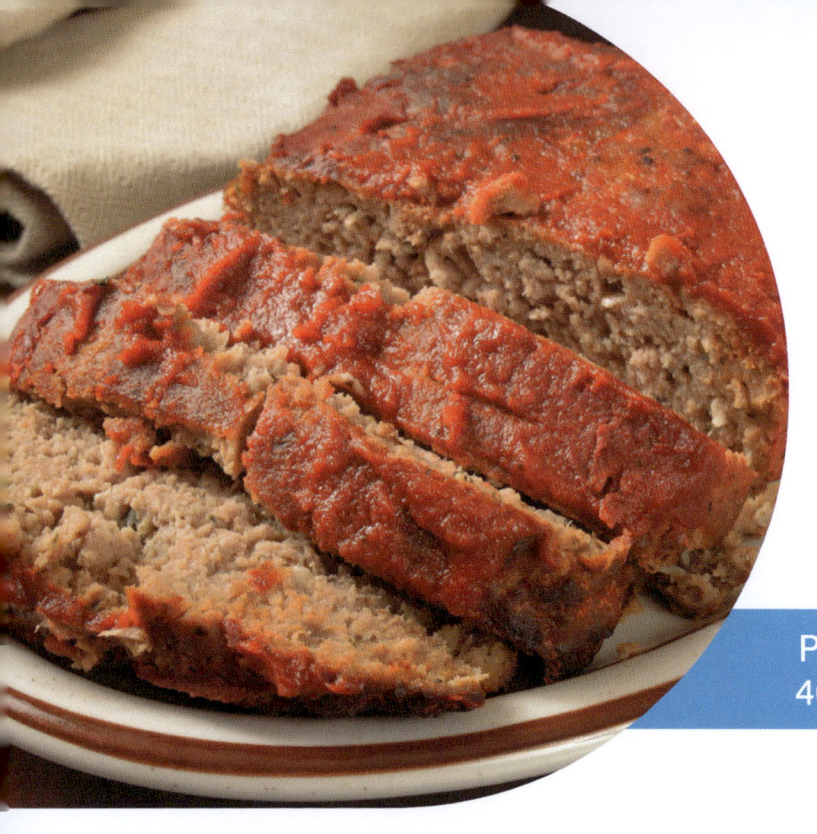

GARLIC PARMESAN TURKEY MEATLOAF

NUTRITION INFORMATION

Calories:	310 Kcal
Protein:	42 g
Carb:	13 g
Fat:	10 g

Prep Time: 40 Minutes	Servings 4

INGREDIENTS

- 1.5 lb ground turkey
- 1/2 cup grated Parmesan cheese
- 1/4 cup breadcrumbs
- 1/4 cup finely chopped onion
- 1/4 cup chopped fresh parsley
- 2 cloves garlic, minced
- 1 large egg, beaten
- 1 tablespoon Worcestershire sauce
- Salt and pepper, to taste

INSTRUCTIONS

1. Combine the ground turkey, Parmesan cheese, breadcrumbs, onion, parsley, garlic, beaten egg, Worcestershire sauce, salt, and pepper in a large mixing bowl. Mix until well combined.
2. Shape the turkey mixture into a loaf on a cutting board or plate. Get the air fryer to a temperature of 375°F (190°C).
3. Carefully place the meatloaf in the air fryer basket. Meatloaf should achieve 165°F (74°C) after 25 minutes. After resting, slice and serve the meatloaf.

CRISPY CHICKPEA TACOS

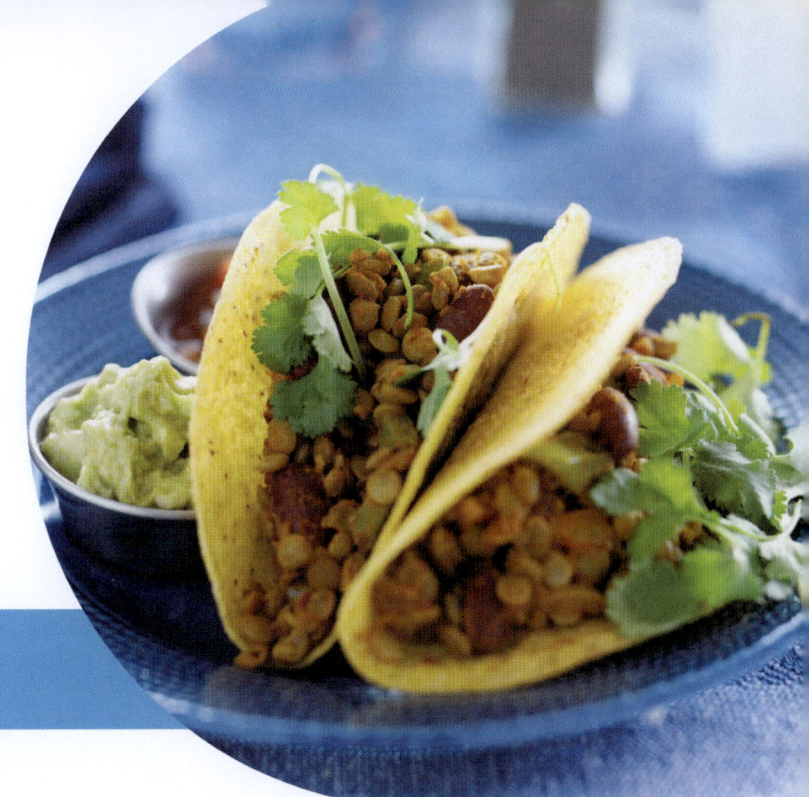

NUTRITION INFORMATION

Calories:	360 Kcal
Protein:	20 g
Carb:	44 g
Fat:	14 g

Prep Time: 25 Minutes	Servings 4

INGREDIENTS

- 1 (15 oz weight) can of chickpeas, drained and rinsed
- 1 tablespoon olive oil
- 1 tablespoon taco seasoning
- ½ teaspoon salt
- 8 small corn tortillas
- 1 cup shredded lettuce
- ½ cup diced tomatoes
- ½ cup shredded cheddar cheese
- ½ cup Greek yogurt

INSTRUCTIONS

1. Toss the chickpeas with olive oil, taco seasoning, and salt in a bowl. Set the air fryer heat to 400°F (200°C). Transfer the seasoned chickpeas to the air fryer basket and cook for 13-15 minutes, shaking the basket halfway through.
2. Warm the tortillas, then assemble the tacos by placing the crispy chickpeas, lettuce, tomatoes, cheese, and a dollop of Greek yogurt on each tortilla. Serve immediately.

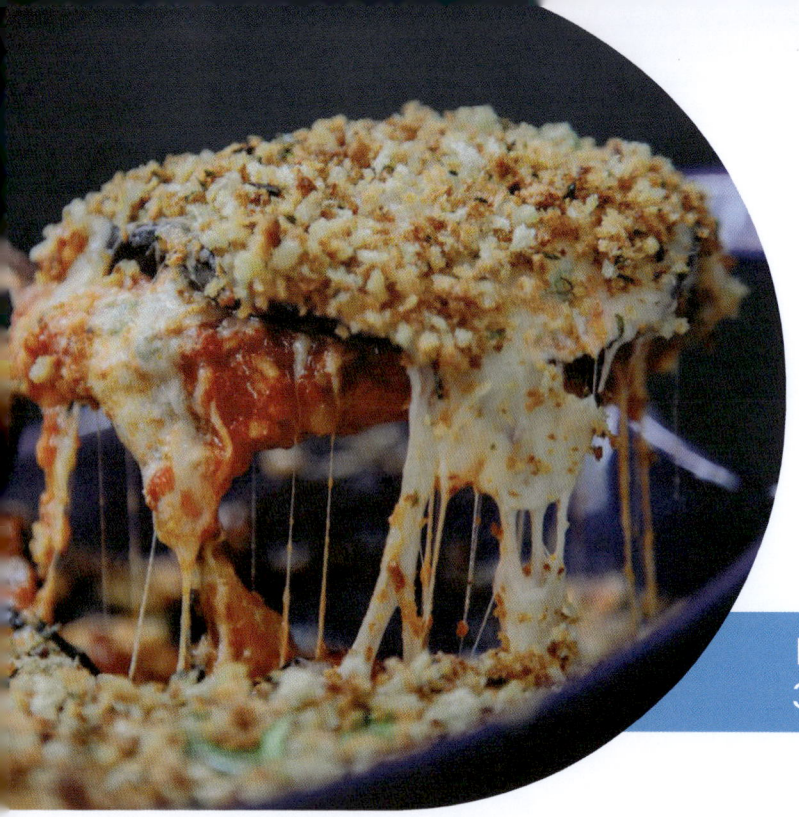

SPICY EGGPLANT PARMESAN

NUTRITION INFORMATION

Calories:	390 Kcal
Protein:	22 g
Carb:	42 g
Fat:	15 g

Prep Time:	Servings
35 Minutes	4

INGREDIENTS

- 1 large eggplant, sliced into ¼-inch rounds
- 1 cup flour
- 2 large eggs, beaten
- 1 cup breadcrumbs
- ½ cup grated Parmesan cheese
- 1 tablespoon Italian seasoning
- ½ teaspoon red pepper flakes
- 1 cup marinara sauce
- 1 cup shredded mozzarella cheese
- Salt and pepper, to taste

INSTRUCTIONS

1. Sprinkle the eggplant slices with salt and crushed pepper. Set up a breading with flour, beaten eggs, and a mixture of breadcrumbs, Parmesan, Italian seasoning, and red pepper flakes. Coat each eggplant slice in flour, dip in beaten eggs, and coat in breadcrumb mixture.
2. Set the air fryer heat to 375°F (190°C). Place the breaded eggplant slices in one layer in the fryer basket and cook for 10 minutes, flipping halfway through. Top each cooked eggplant slice with marinara sauce and mozzarella cheese, then cook for another 10 minutes.
3. Serve immediately.

STUFFED ZUCCHINI BOATS

NUTRITION INFORMATION

Calories:	400 Kcal
Protein:	28 g
Carb:	37 g
Fat:	15 g

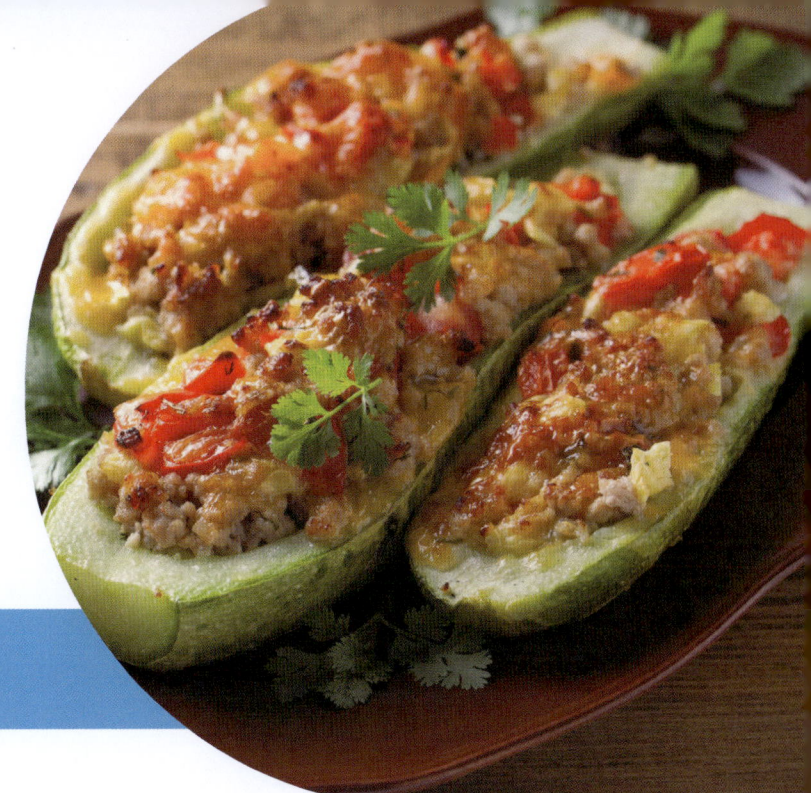

Prep Time: 35 Minutes	Servings 4

INGREDIENTS

- 4 medium zucchini
- 1 lb. lean ground turkey
- ½ cup chopped onion
- 2 cloves garlic, minced
- 1 cup marinara sauce
- 1 cup cooked quinoa
- ½ cup shredded mozzarella cheese
- Salt and pepper, to taste

INSTRUCTIONS

1. Cut the zucchini lengthwise to scoop the seeds to create a boat-like shape. Season with salt and pepper. In a skillet, cook the ground turkey, onion, and garlic until the turkey is browned and cooked. Drain any excess liquid.
2. Stir in the marinara sauce and cooked quinoa, then powder with salt and crushed pepper to taste. Set the air fryer heat to 350°F (175°C). Spoon the turkey and quinoa mixture into the zucchini boats, then top each with shredded mozzarella cheese.
3. Place the stuffed zucchini boats in the air fryer basket and cook for 20 minutes until the zucchini is tender. Serve immediately.

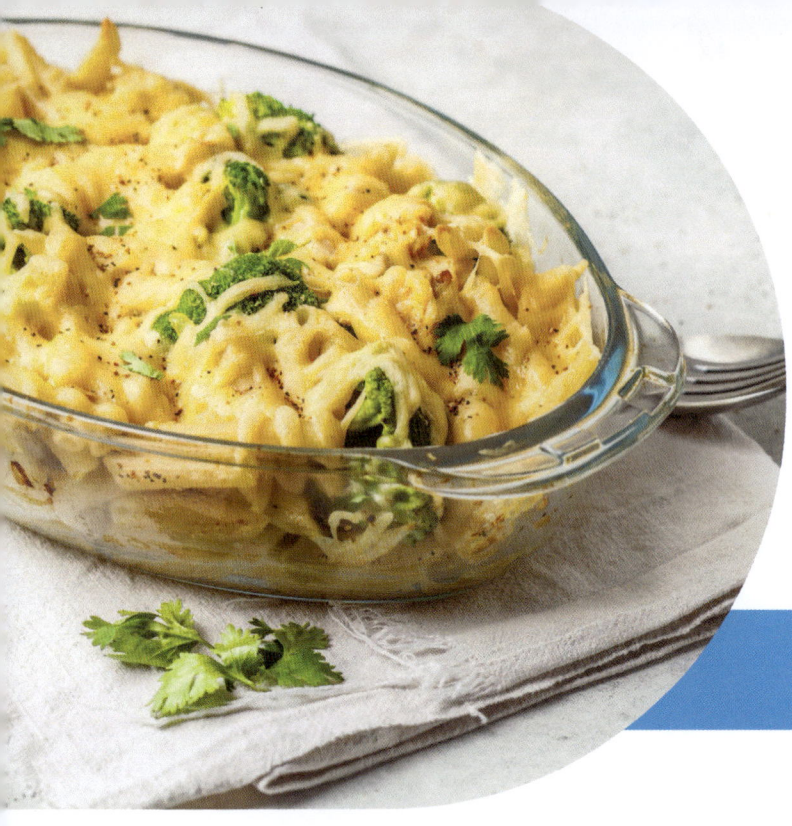

CHEESY CAULIFLOWER AND BROCCOLI BAKE

NUTRITION INFORMATION

Calories:	200 Kcal
Protein:	20 g
Carb:	10 g
Fat:	10 g

Prep Time:	Servings
25 Minutes	4

INGREDIENTS

- 2 cups cauliflower florets
- 2 cups broccoli florets
- 1 cup shredded cheddar cheese
- ½ cup Greek yogurt
- ¼ cup grated Parmesan cheese
- ¼ teaspoon garlic powder
- ¼ teaspoon onion powder
- Salt and pepper, to taste

INSTRUCTIONS

1. Combine the cauliflower, broccoli, cheddar cheese, Greek yogurt, Parmesan cheese, garlic, onion powder, salt, and pepper in a large bowl. Set the air fryer heat to 350°F (175°C). Transfer the cauliflower and broccoli mixture to an air-fryer-safe baking dish or pan.
2. Cook for 13-15 minutes or until the vegetables are tender. Serve immediately.

LEMON HERB QUINOA STUFFED TOMATOES

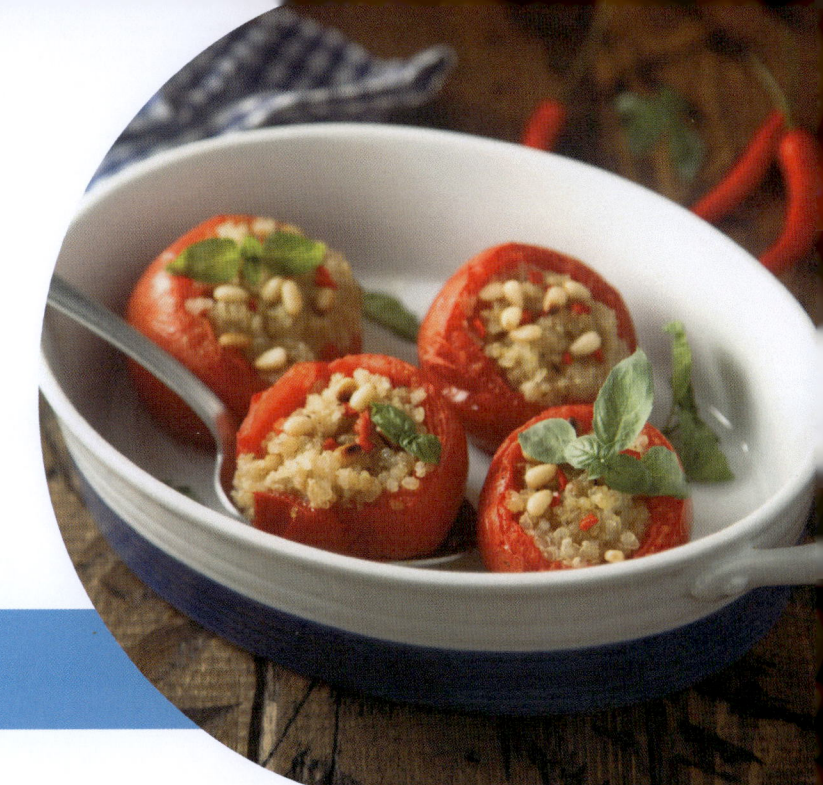

NUTRITION INFORMATION

Calories:	290 Kcal
Protein:	21 g
Carb:	38 g
Fat:	8 g

Prep Time: 247 Minutes	Servings 4

INGREDIENTS

- 4 large tomatoes
- 2 cups cooked quinoa
- ¼ cup crumbled feta cheese
- ¼ cup chopped fresh parsley
- 2 tablespoons chopped fresh basil
- 2 tablespoons lemon juice
- 1 tablespoon olive oil
- Salt and pepper, to taste

INSTRUCTIONS

1. Cut the tomatoes tops and scoop out the seeds and pulp, creating a hollow cavity. Season with salt and pepper. Combine the cooked quinoa, feta cheese, parsley, basil, lemon juice, olive oil, salt, and crushed pepper in a bowl.
2. Spoon the quinoa mixture into the hollowed-out tomatoes, packing it in tightly. Set the air fryer heat to 350°F (175°C). Place the stuffed tomatoes in the air fryer basket and cook for 11-12 minutes until the tomatoes are tender and the quinoa filling is heated.
3. Serve immediately.

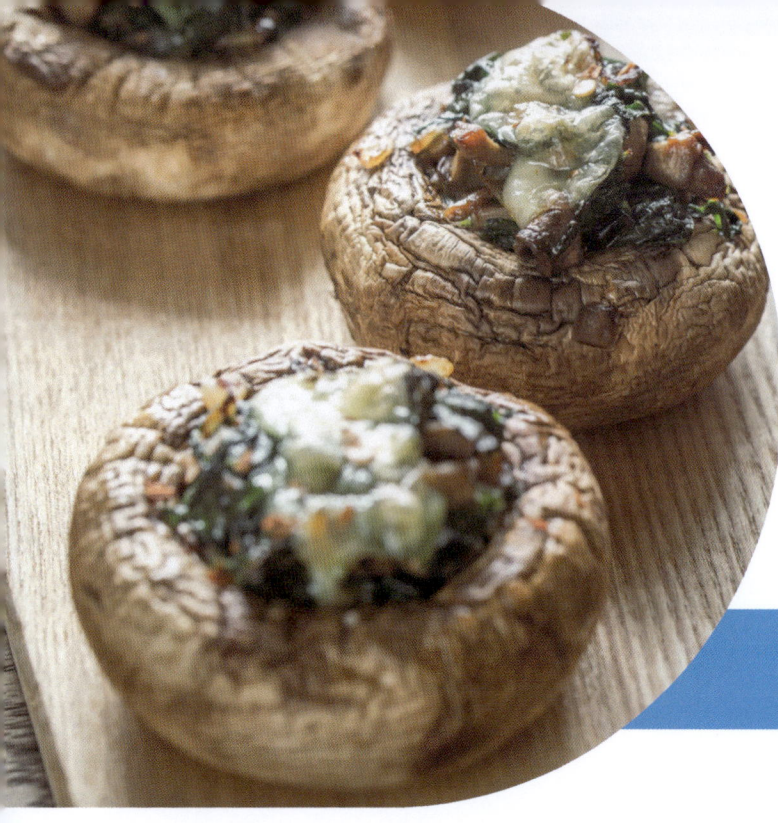

SPINACH AND FETA STUFFED PORTOBELLO MUSHROOMS

NUTRITION INFORMATION

Calories:	170 Kcal
Protein:	20 g
Carb:	8 g
Fat:	9 g

Prep Time: 30 Minutes	Servings 4

INGREDIENTS

- 4 large portobello mushroom caps
- 3 cups chopped fresh spinach
- ¾ cup crumbled feta cheese
- ¼ cup finely chopped red onion
- 1 clove garlic, minced
- 1 tablespoon olive oil
- Salt and pepper, to taste

INSTRUCTIONS

1. Clean the portobello mushroom caps and remove the stems. Combine the chopped spinach, feta cheese, red onion, garlic, olive oil, salt, and pepper in a bowl. Spoon the spinach mixture into the mushroom caps, pressing down to fill each cap evenly.
2. Set the air fryer heat to 350°F (175°C). Place the stuffed mushroom caps in the air fryer basket and cook for 15 minutes until the mushrooms are tender. Serve immediately.

CAPRESE STUFFED CHICKEN

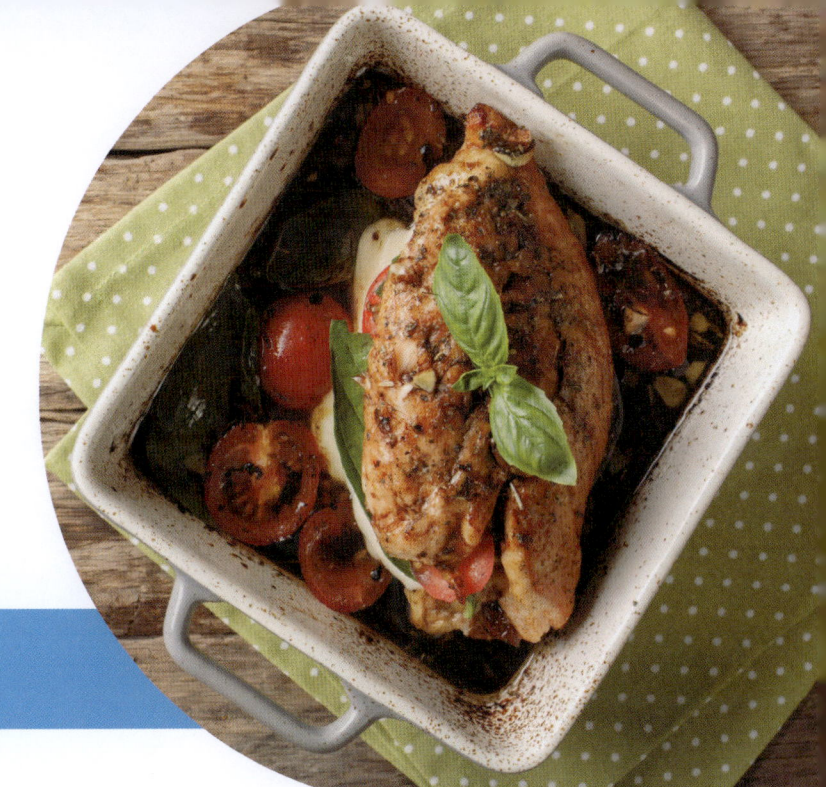

NUTRITION INFORMATION

Calories:	310 Kcal
Protein:	28 g
Carb:	11 g
Fat:	10 g

Prep Time: 35 Minutes	Servings 4

INGREDIENTS

- 4 boneless, skinless chicken breasts
- 1 cup cherry tomatoes, halved
- ½ cup fresh basil leaves, chopped
- ¾ cup shredded mozzarella cheese
- ¼ cup grated Parmesan cheese
- 2 tablespoons balsamic glaze
- Salt and pepper, to taste

INSTRUCTIONS

1. Cut a pocket in each chicken breast, careful not to cut all the way through. Combine the cherry tomatoes, basil leaves, mozzarella cheese, and Parmesan cheese in a bowl. Stuff the chicken pockets with the tomato mixture, then secure the openings with toothpicks.
2. Season the stuffed chicken breasts with salt and pepper. Set the air fryer heat to 375°F (190°C). Cook the chicken breasts in the air fryer basket for 20 minutes or until the internal temperature reaches 165°F (74°C).
3. Drizzle the cooked chicken with balsamic glaze and serve.

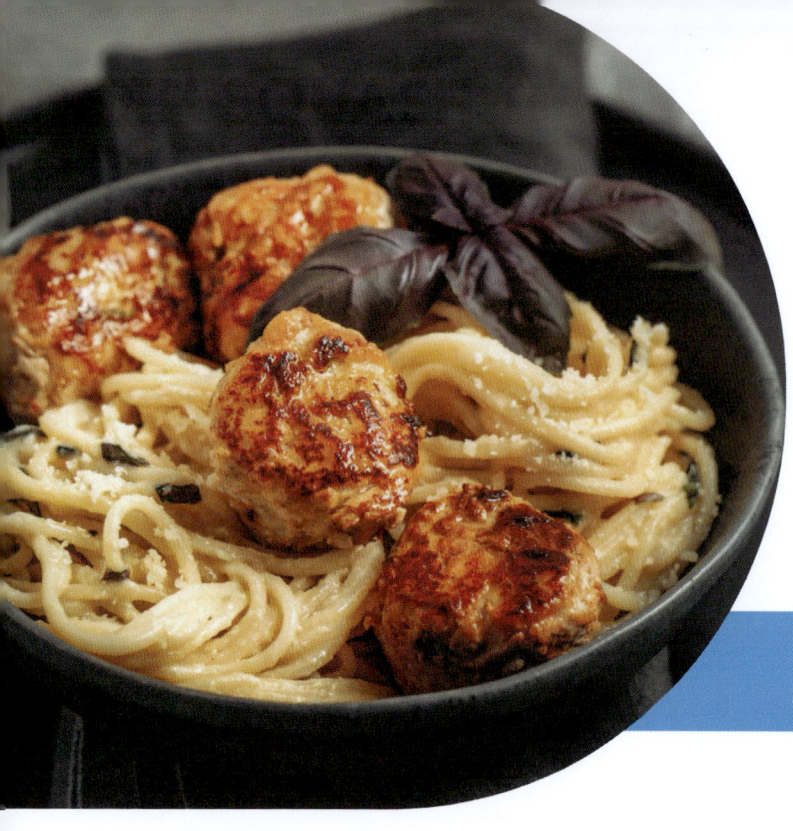

SPAGHETTI SQUASH AND TURKEY MEATBALLS

NUTRITION INFORMATION

Calories:	410 Kcal
Protein:	27 g
Carb:	39 g
Fat:	17 g

Prep Time: 50 Minutes	Servings 4

INGREDIENTS

- 1 spaghetti squash, halved and seedless
- 1 lb. lean ground turkey
- ¼ cup breadcrumbs
- ¼ cup grated Parmesan cheese
- ¼ cup chopped fresh parsley
- 1 large egg, beaten
- 2 cloves garlic, minced
- ½ teaspoon salt
- ¼ teaspoon black pepper
- 1½ cups marinara sauce

INSTRUCTIONS

1. Set the air fryer heat to 370°F (190°C). Put the spaghetti squash halves cut side down in the fryer basket and cook for 27-30 minutes or until the flesh is tender.
2. While the spaghetti squash is cooking, combine the ground turkey, breadcrumbs, Parmesan cheese, parsley, egg, garlic, salt, and black pepper in a bowl. Mix well and form 16 small meatballs.
3. Set the air fryer heat to 400°F (200°C). Cook the meatball for 13-15 minutes until cooked thoroughly. Meanwhile, heat the marinara sauce in a saucepan over medium heat.
4. When the spaghetti squash is cooked, use a fork/butter knife to scrape the flesh into spaghetti-like strands. Serve the spaghetti squash topped with the turkey meatballs and marinara sauce.

SWEET POTATO AND BLACK BEAN QUESADILLAS

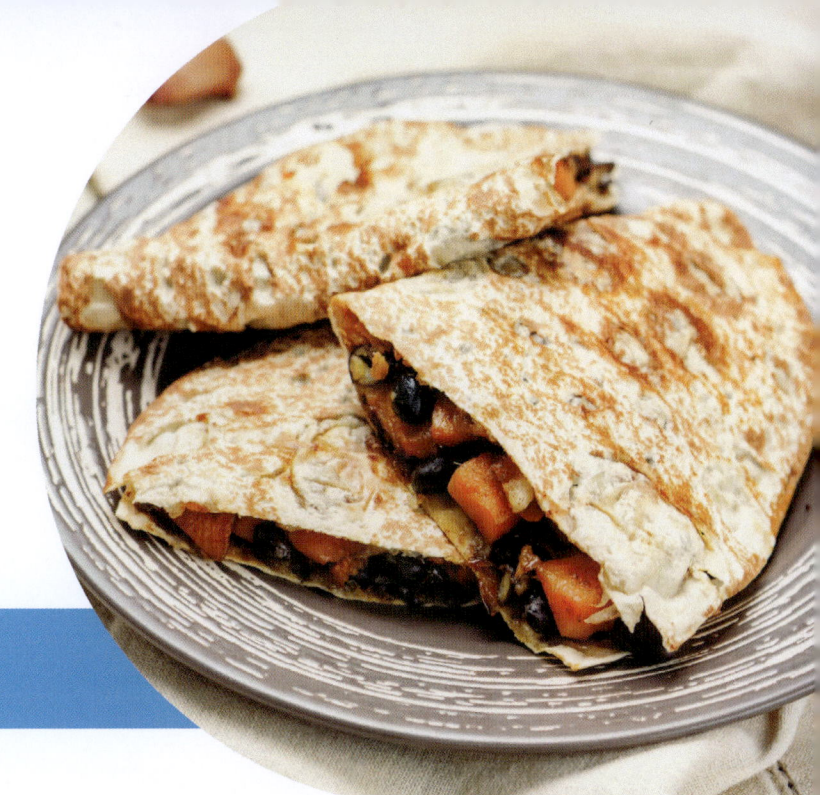

NUTRITION INFORMATION

Calories:	480 Kcal
Protein:	21 g
Carb:	62 g
Fat:	17 g

Prep Time: 30 Minutes	Servings 4

INGREDIENTS

- 2 medium sweet potatoes, cooked and mashed
- 1 cup cooked/canned black beans, drained and rinsed
- 1 cup shredded cheddar cheese
- ½ cup chopped green onions
- ½ teaspoon cumin
- ¼ teaspoon chili powder
- Salt and pepper, to taste
- 8 small flour tortillas

INSTRUCTIONS

1. Combine the mashed sweet potatoes, black beans, cheddar cheese, green onions, cumin, chili powder, salt, and pepper in a bowl. Spread the mixture evenly over 4 tortillas, then top each with another tortilla.
2. Set the air fryer heat to 360°F (180°C). Cook the quesadillas in the air fryer basket for 6 minutes for each side or until golden brown and crispy. Cut the quesadillas into 6 or 8 wedges and serve with your favorite dipping sauce.

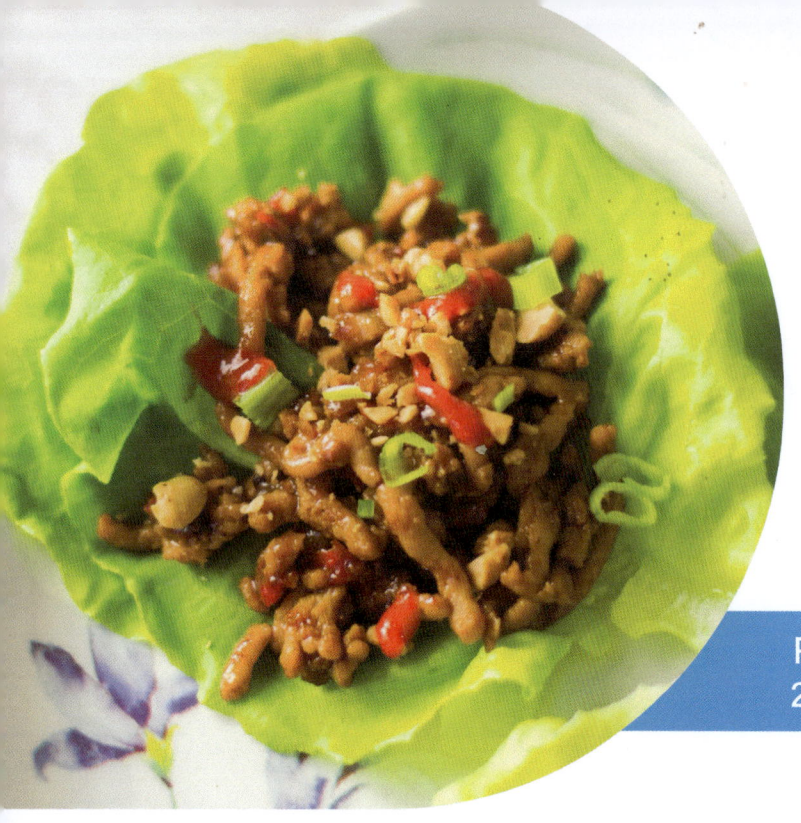

THAI TURKEY LETTUCE WRAPS

NUTRITION INFORMATION

Calories:	230 Kcal
Protein:	25 g
Carb:	14 g
Fat:	8 g

Prep Time:	Servings
25 Minutes	4

INGREDIENTS

- 1 lb. lean ground turkey
- ¼ cup chopped fresh cilantro
- ¼ cup chopped green/spring onions
- ¼ cup chopped red bell pepper
- 2 cloves garlic, minced
- 2 tablespoons soy sauce

- 1 tablespoon fish sauce
- 1 tablespoon lime juice
- 1 tablespoon honey
- ½ teaspoon red pepper flakes (optional)
- 1 head of butter lettuce, leaves separated and washed

INSTRUCTIONS

1. In a non-stick skillet, cook the ground turkey over medium heat until browned and cooked, breaking it into small pieces as it cooks. Add cilantro, green onions, red bell pepper, and garlic, and cook for three minutes until the veggies are softened.
2. In a bowl, whisk the soy sauce with fish sauce, lime juice, honey, and crushed red pepper flakes (if using). Pour the sauce over the turkey mixture in the skillet and cook for 2-3 minutes, stirring to combine.
3. Set the air fryer heat to 400°F (200°C). Place a few spoonfuls of the turkey mixture onto each lettuce leaf, then fold the leaves in half to form a wrap. Arrange the lettuce wraps in one layer in the fryer basket and cook for 5-6 minutes until the lettuce is slightly wilted and the filling is heated.
4. Immediately serve the Thai turkey lettuce wraps and top with cilantro and green/spring onions if desired.

VEGAN LENTIL BURGERS

NUTRITION INFORMATION

Calories:	290 Kcal
Protein:	21 g
Carb:	40 g
Fat:	5 g

Prep Time: 30 Minutes	Servings 4

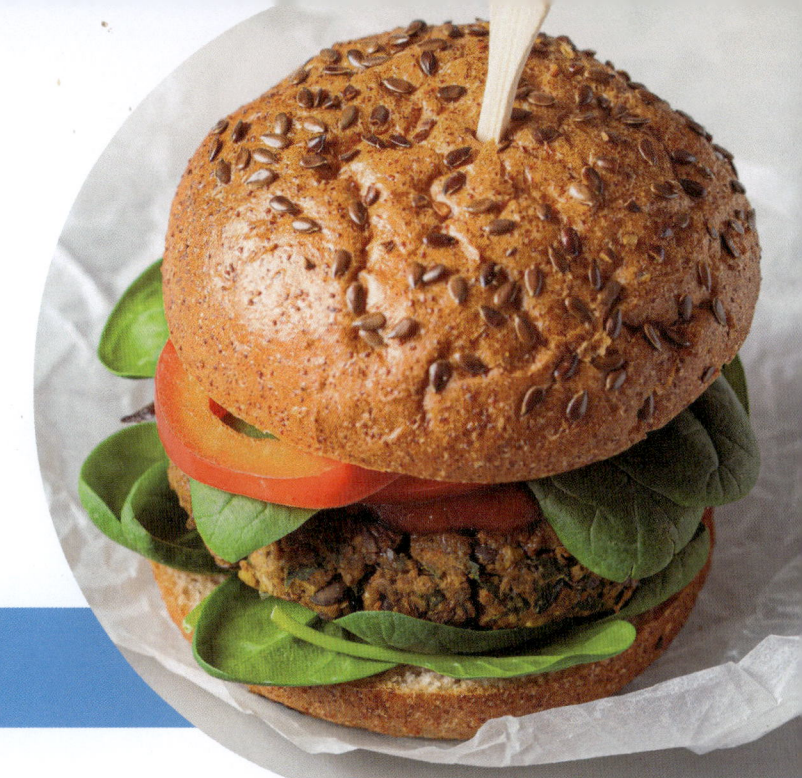

INGREDIENTS

- 1 can (15 oz) of cooked lentils, drained and rinsed
- ½ cup breadcrumbs
- ¼ cup chopped onion
- 2 cloves garlic, minced
- 2 tablespoons chopped fresh parsley
- 2 tablespoons ground flaxseed
- 2 tablespoons water
- 1 tablespoon soy sauce
- ½ teaspoon smoked paprika
- Salt and pepper, to taste

INSTRUCTIONS

1. Combine the cooked lentils, breadcrumbs, onion, garlic, parsley, flaxseed, water, soy sauce, smoked paprika, salt, and pepper in a large bowl. Mix well. Use your hands to form the lentil mixture into 4 equal-sized patties.
2. Set the air fryer heat to 375°F (190°C). Place the lentil patties in the fryer basket and cook for 11-12 minutes, flipping halfway through, until they are browned and crispy. Serve the lentil burgers on buns with your favorite toppings.

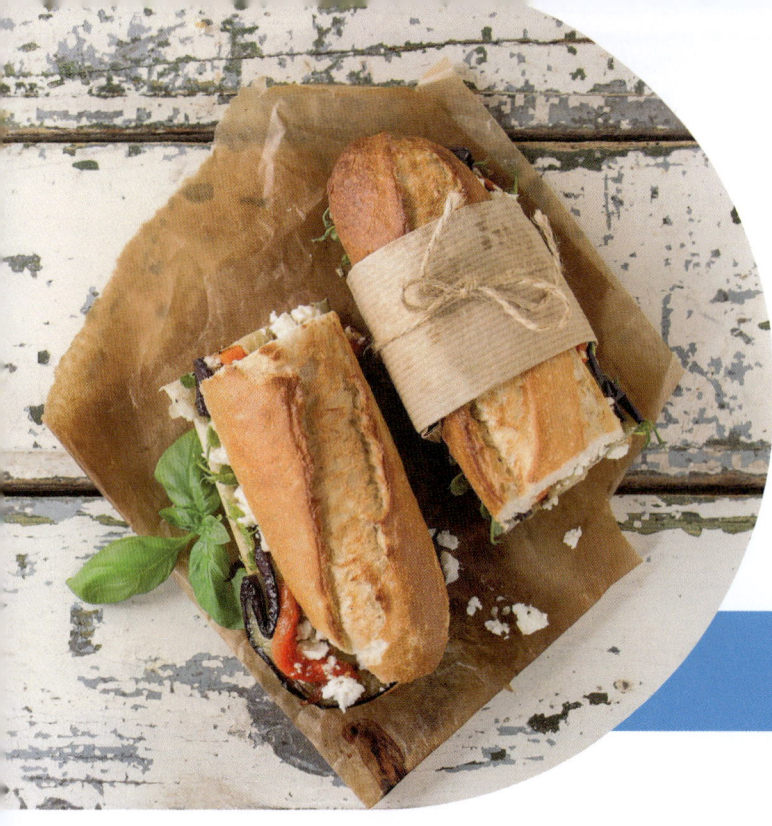

VEGETARIAN EGGPLANT ROLLATINI

NUTRITION INFORMATION

Calories:	140 Kcal
Protein:	21 g
Carb:	15 g
Fat:	6 g

Prep Time:	Servings
40 Minutes	4

INGREDIENTS

- 1 large eggplant, sliced lengthwise into 8 thin slices
- 1 cup part-skim ricotta cheese
- ¼ cup chopped fresh basil
- ½ cup grated Parmesan cheese
- 1 clove garlic, minced
- Salt and pepper, to taste
- 1 cup marinara sauce

INSTRUCTIONS

1. Set the air fryer heat to 375°F (190°C). Mix the ricotta cheese, basil, Parmesan cheese, garlic, salt, and pepper in a bowl. Lay the eggplant slices flat and spoon the ricotta mixture onto each slice.
2. Roll up each slice of eggplant and place seam-side down in the air fryer basket. Cook the eggplant rollatini in the air fryer for 20 minutes until the eggplant is tender and the filling is heated.
3. Serve the eggplant rollatini with marinara sauce.

BAKED SPINACH AND RICOTTA STUFFED SHELLS

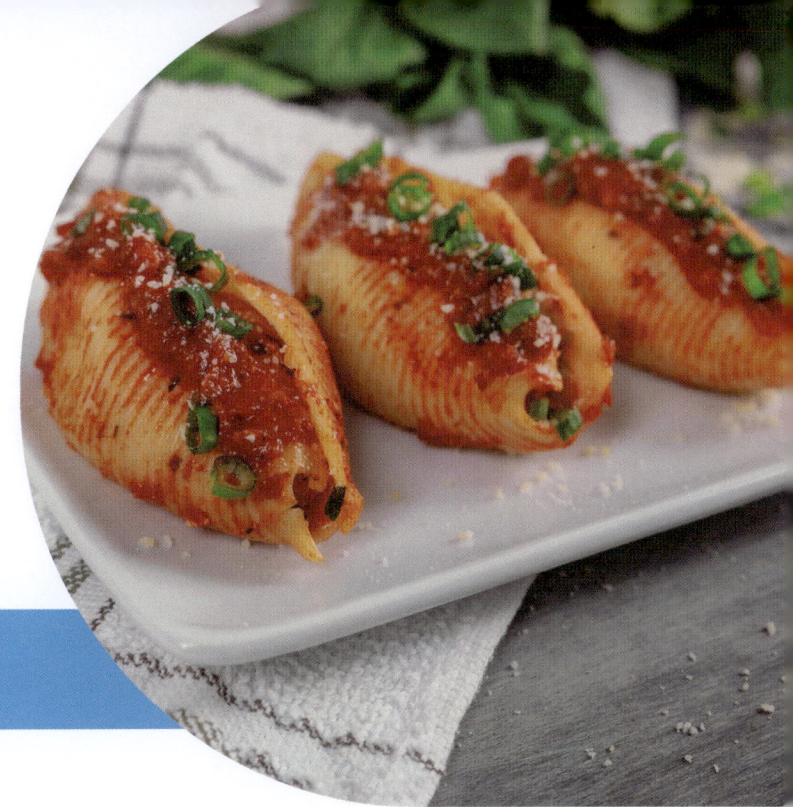

NUTRITION INFORMATION

Calories:	290 Kcal
Protein:	21 g
Carb:	38 g
Fat:	6 g

Prep Time: 38 Minutes	Servings 4

INGREDIENTS

- 12 jumbo pasta shells, cooked according to package instructions
- 1 cup part-skim ricotta cheese
- ½ cup chopped frozen spinach, thawed and drained
- ¼ cup grated Parmesan cheese
- ¼ teaspoon garlic powder
- Salt and pepper, to taste
- 1 cup marinara sauce

INSTRUCTIONS

1. Set the air fryer heat to 375°F (190°C). Mix the ricotta, spinach, Parmesan, and garlic powder in a bowl. Add salt and pepper to taste. Stuff each cooked pasta shell with the ricotta mixture.
2. Place the stuffed shells in the air fryer basket and cook for 18 minutes until the shells are heated, and the tops are slightly browned. Serve the stuffed shells with marinara sauce.

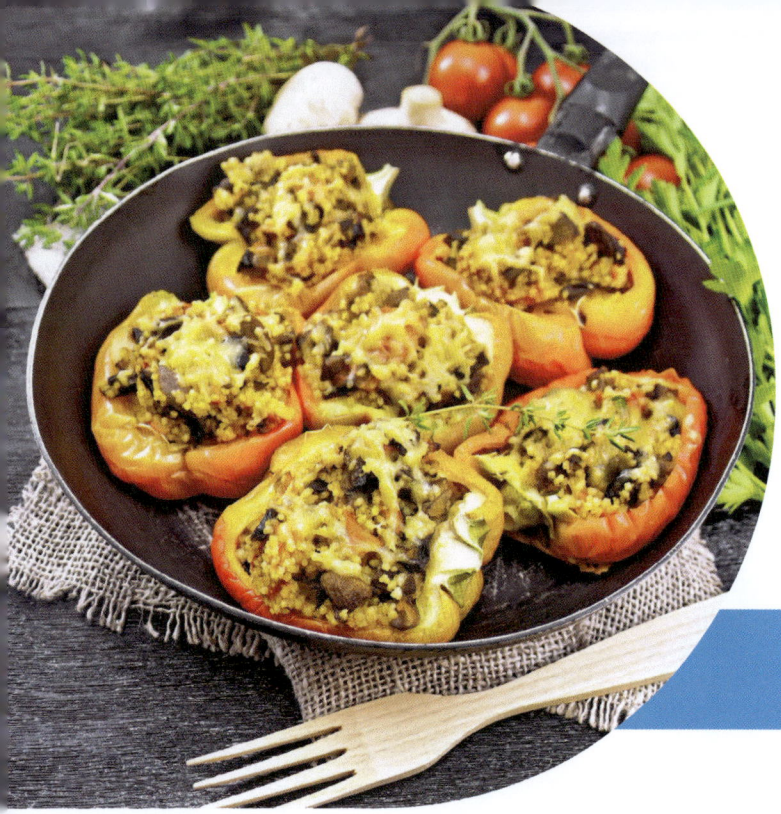

CHEESY MUSHROOM AND QUINOA STUFFED PEPPERS

NUTRITION INFORMATION

Calories:	376 Kcal
Protein:	22 g
Carb:	36 g
Fat:	16 g

Prep Time: 40 Minutes	Servings 4

INGREDIENTS

- 4 large bell peppers, halved and seeded
- 1 cup cooked quinoa
- 1 cup chopped mushrooms
- 2 cups shredded cheddar cheese
- ¼ cup chopped onion
- 1 clove garlic, minced
- Salt and pepper, to taste

INSTRUCTIONS

1. Set the air fryer heat to 375°F (190°C). Mix the cooked quinoa, mushrooms, cheddar cheese, onion, garlic, salt, and pepper in a bowl. Stuff each pepper half with the quinoa mixture. Put the stuffed peppers in the fryer basket and cook for 18 minutes until the peppers are tender.
2. Serve the stuffed peppers as a main dish or a side dish.

GREEK FALAFEL PITAS

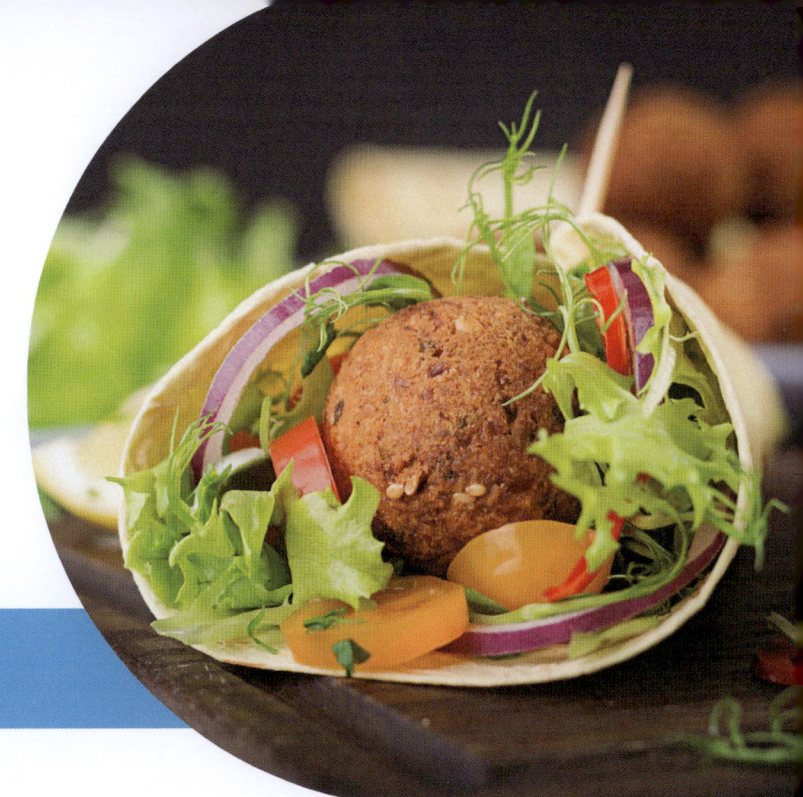

NUTRITION INFORMATION

Calories:	367 Kcal
Protein:	23 g
Carb:	53 g
Fat:	7 g

Prep Time: 30 Minutes	Servings 4

INGREDIENTS

- 2 cans (15 oz) of chickpeas, drained and rinsed
- 1/2 cup chopped fresh parsley
- 1/4 cup chopped fresh cilantro
- 1/4 cup chopped onion
- 1/4 cup breadcrumbs
- 1 clove garlic, minced
- 2 tablespoons lemon juice
- 1 teaspoon ground cumin
- 1/2 teaspoon salt
- 4 whole wheat pita bread
- 1/2 cup tzatziki sauce

INSTRUCTIONS

1. In a food processor, combine chickpeas, parsley, cilantro, onion, breadcrumbs, garlic, lemon juice, cumin, and salt. Pulse until the mixture is coarsely chopped. Set the air fryer heat to 375°F (190°C). Shape the chickpea mixture into small balls.
2. Put the falafel balls in the fryer basket and cook for 10 minutes until they are browned and crispy. Warm the pita bread in the air fryer for 1-2 minutes.
3. Serve the falafel balls on the pita bread with tzatziki sauce.

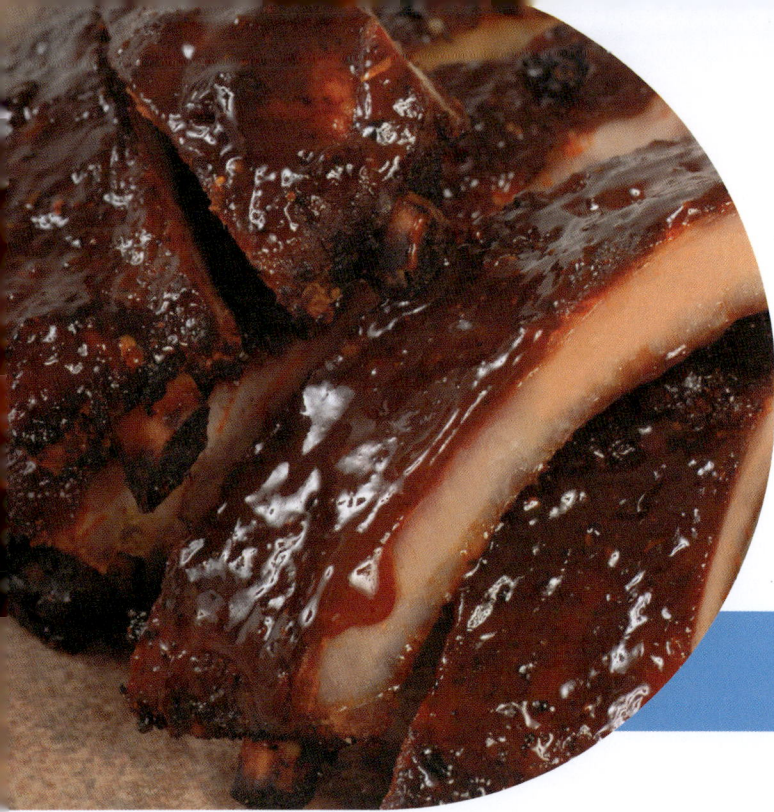

BAKED BBQ TEMPEH

NUTRITION INFORMATION

Calories:	396 Kcal
Protein:	22 g
Carb:	25 g
Fat:	12 g

Prep Time: 22 Minutes	Servings 4

INGREDIENTS

- 2 packets (8 oz each weight) of tempeh, sliced
- ½ cup barbecue sauce
- 1 tablespoon olive oil

INSTRUCTIONS

1. Set the air fryer heat to 375°F (190°C). In a bowl, mix the barbecue sauce and olive oil. Add the tempeh slices to the bowl and toss to coat evenly. Place the tempeh slices in the fryer basket and cook for 11-12 minutes, flipping halfway through.
2. Serve the baked BBQ tempeh as a main dish or a sandwich filling.

SPICY TOFU AND PINEAPPLE SKEWERS

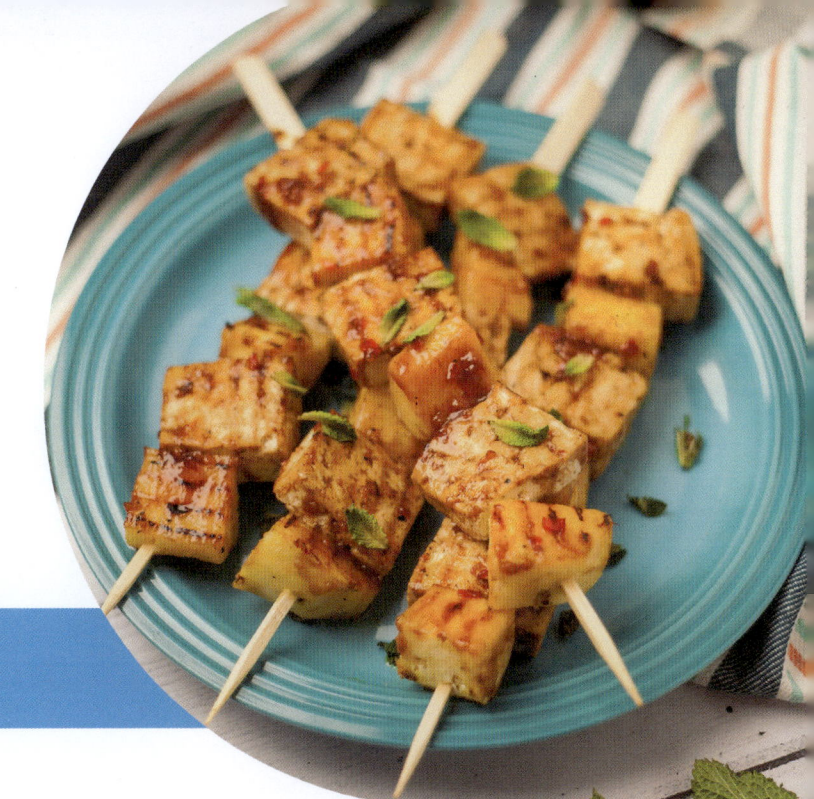

NUTRITION INFORMATION

Calories:	281 Kcal
Protein:	21 g
Carb:	20 g
Fat:	13 g

Prep Time: 25 Minutes	Servings 4

INGREDIENTS

- 2 packets (14 oz each weight) of firm tofu, cut into cubes
- 1 cup fresh pineapple chunks
- 2 tablespoons soy sauce
- 1 tablespoon hot sauce
- 1 tablespoon honey
- 1 tablespoon olive oil
- 1 teaspoon smoked paprika
- ½ teaspoon garlic powder
- 8 wooden skewers, soaked for 30 minutes in water

INSTRUCTIONS

1. Mix the soy sauce, hot sauce, honey, olive oil, smoked paprika powder, and garlic powder in a bowl. Add tofu and pineapple chunks to the marinade and toss to coat evenly. Cover and refrigerate for 30 minutes.
2. Set the air fryer heat to 375°F (190°C). Thread the marinated tofu and pineapple onto the soaked wooden skewers. Put the skewers in the fryer basket, ensuring they do not touch. Cook the skewers for 10 minutes, flipping halfway through, until they are browned and crispy.
3. Serve the spicy tofu and pineapple skewers as a main dish or appetizer.

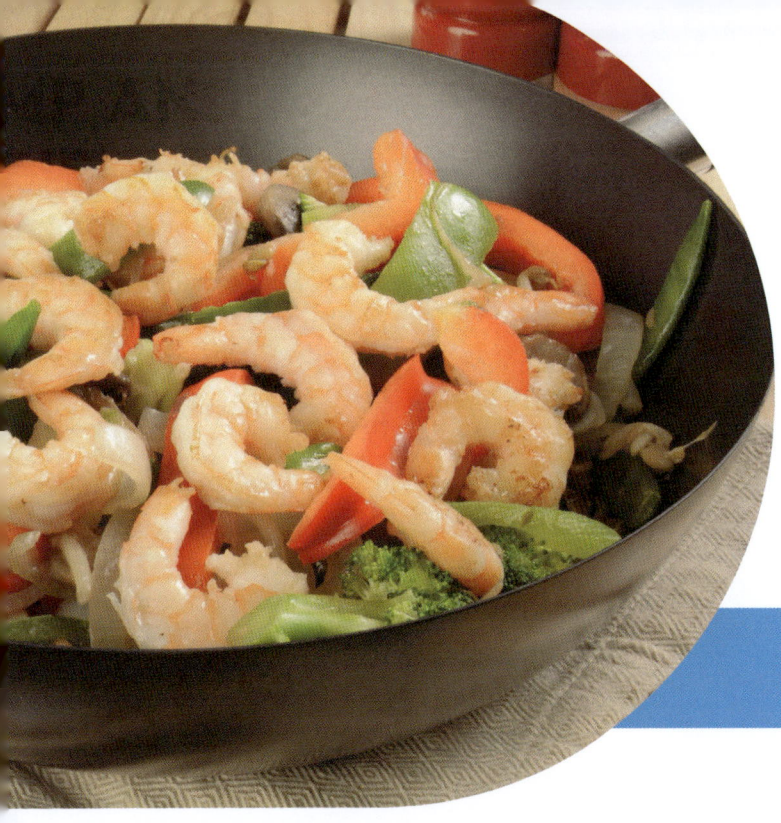

SHRIMP AND VEGGIE STIR-FRY

NUTRITION INFORMATION

Calories:	170 Kcal
Protein:	21 g
Carb:	14 g
Fat:	4 g

Prep Time:	Servings
25 Minutes	4

INGREDIENTS

- 1 lb. large shrimp, peeled and deveined
- 1 cup chopped broccoli florets
- 1 cup sliced bell peppers
- 1 cup sliced onions
- 2 tablespoons soy sauce
- 1 tablespoon honey
- 1 tablespoon sesame oil
- ½ teaspoon garlic powder
- Salt and pepper, to taste

INSTRUCTIONS

1. Set the air fryer heat to 375°F (190°C). Whisk the soy sauce, honey, sesame oil, garlic powder, salt, and pepper in a bowl. Add shrimp, broccoli, bell peppers, and onions to the bowl and toss to coat evenly.
2. Place the shrimp and vegetables in the air fryer basket and cook for 10 minutes, stirring halfway through, until the shrimp is done thoroughly and the vegetables are tender.
3. Serve the shrimp and veggie stir-fry over a bed of rice or quinoa or as a standalone dish.

CHICKEN AND VEGGIE FAJITA WRAPS

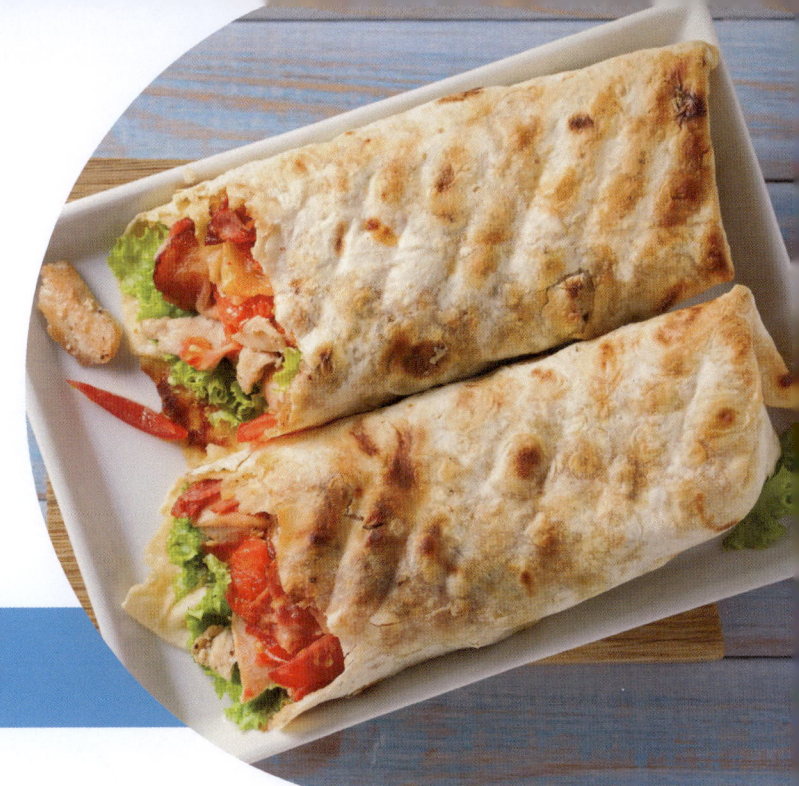

NUTRITION INFORMATION

Calories:	370 Kcal
Protein:	25 g
Carb:	38 g
Fat:	14 g

Prep Time: 30 Minutes	Servings 4

INGREDIENTS

- 1 lb. chicken breasts without skin & bone, sliced
- 1 red bell pepper, sliced
- 1 green bell pepper, sliced
- 1 yellow onion, sliced
- 2 tablespoons olive oil
- 1 tablespoon chili powder
- 1 teaspoon smoked paprika
- 1 teaspoon garlic powder
- Salt and pepper, to taste
- 4 whole wheat tortillas

INSTRUCTIONS

1. Set the air fryer heat to 375°F (190°C). Mix the olive oil, chili powder, smoked paprika, garlic powder, salt, and pepper. Add the chicken, bell peppers, and onion to the bowl and toss to coat evenly.
2. Place the chicken and veggies in the air fryer basket and cook for 15 minutes, stirring halfway through, until the chicken is cooked and the veggies are tender and lightly charred. Warm the tortillas in the air fryer for 1-2 minutes.
3. Divide the chicken and veggie mixture evenly among the tortillas and roll them up tightly. Serve the fajita wraps with salsa and guacamole if desired.

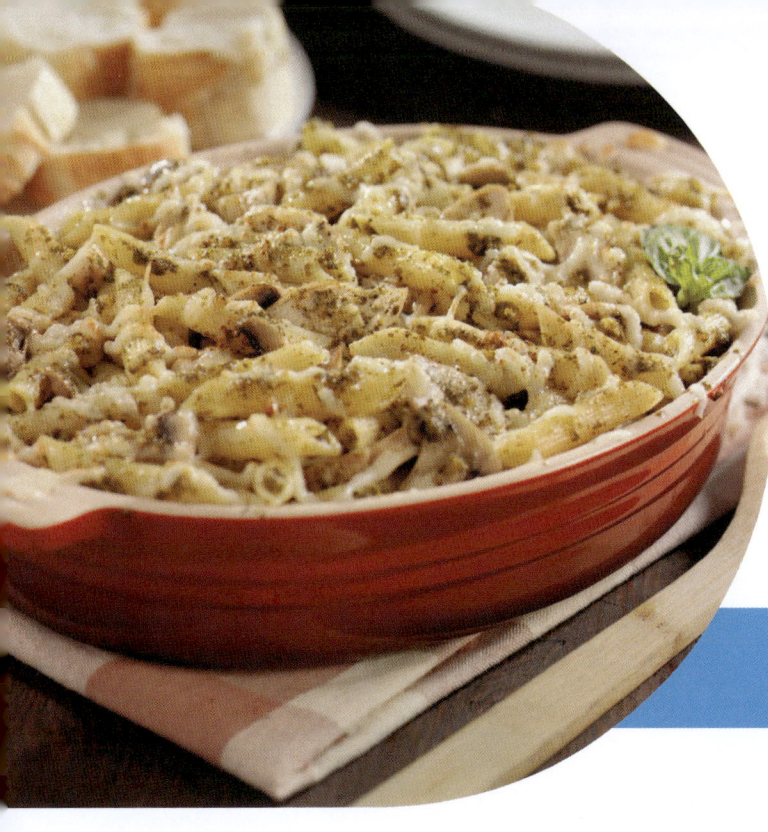

CREAMY PESTO CHICKEN AND VEGGIE BAKE

NUTRITION INFORMATION

Calories:	350 Kcal
Protein:	23 g
Carb:	10 g
Fat:	24 g

Prep Time: 35 Minutes	Servings 4

INGREDIENTS

- 1 lb. boneless, skinless chicken breasts, sliced
- 2 cups sliced zucchini
- 1 cup cherry tomatoes, halved
- 1/2 cup basil pesto
- 1/4 cup heavy cream
- Salt and pepper, to taste
- 1/4 cup shredded Parmesan cheese

INSTRUCTIONS

1. Set the air fryer heat to 375°F (190°C). In a bowl, whisk the basil pesto with heavy cream. Add chicken, zucchini, and cherry tomatoes to the bowl and toss to coat evenly. Place the chicken and veggies in the air fryer basket and cook for 19-20 minutes, stirring halfway through, until the chicken is cooked and the veggies are tender.
2. Sprinkle shredded Parmesan cheese over the chicken and veggies and cook for 2-3 minutes until the cheese is melted and bubbly. Serve the creamy pesto chicken and veggie bake as a standalone dish or over a bed of pasta or rice.

BLACKENED TOFU TACOS

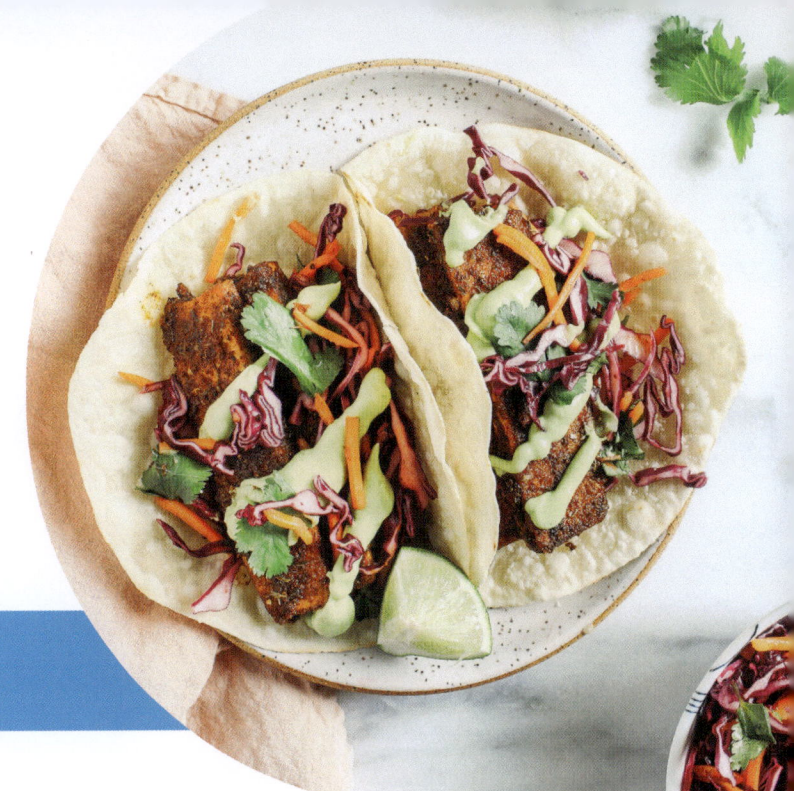

NUTRITION INFORMATION

Calories:	363 Kcal
Protein:	22 g
Carb:	35 g
Fat:	15 g

Prep Time:	Servings
20 Minutes	4

INGREDIENTS

- 2 blocks of extra firm tofu, sliced
- 1 tablespoon olive oil
- 1 tablespoon smoked paprika
- 1 teaspoon garlic powder
- 1/2 teaspoon salt
- 1/4 teaspoon black pepper
- 8 corn tortillas
- Toppings: shredded lettuce, diced tomatoes, sliced avocado, hot sauce

INSTRUCTIONS

1. Whisk the olive oil with smoked paprika, garlic powder, salt, and crushed black pepper in a small bowl. Add sliced tofu to the marinade and toss to coat evenly. Cover and refrigerate for 30 minutes.
2. Set the air fryer heat to 400°F (200°C). Place the marinated tofu in the fryer basket and cook for 7-10 minutes; flip after halftime until the tofu is crispy and blackened. Warm the corn tortillas in the air fryer for 1-2 minutes.
3. Assemble the tacos with the blackened tofu and desired toppings.

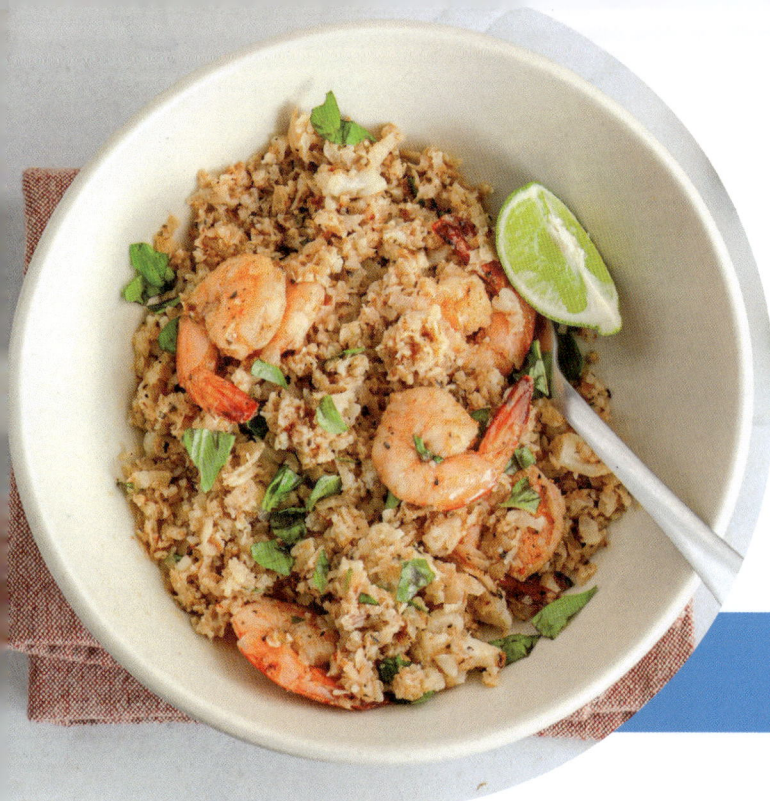

CAULIFLOWER FRIED RICE WITH SHRIMP

NUTRITION INFORMATION

Calories:	220 Kcal
Protein:	22 g
Carb:	12 g
Fat:	10 g

Prep Time: 30 Minutes	Servings 4

INGREDIENTS

- 1 head of cauliflower, grated
- 1 lb. shrimp, peeled and deveined
- 2 tablespoons olive oil
- 1 tablespoon soy sauce
- 1 tablespoon sesame oil
- 2 cloves garlic, minced
- 1/2 teaspoon ground ginger
- Salt and pepper, to taste
- 2 eggs, whisked
- 1/4 cup chopped scallions

INSTRUCTIONS

1. Set the air fryer heat to 375°F (190°C). Mix the olive oil, soy sauce, sesame oil, garlic, ginger, salt, and pepper in a bowl. Add shrimp to the bowl and toss to coat evenly. Put the shrimp in the fryer basket and cook for 5-7 minutes until the shrimp are pink and cooked.
2. Remove the shrimp from the fryer and set aside. In a large non-stick skillet, heat some oil over medium heat. Add the whisked eggs and scramble until cooked through. Remove from the skillet and set aside.
3. In the same skillet, add the grated cauliflower and sauté for 5-7 minutes, until tender and lightly browned.
4. Add the cooked shrimp and scrambled eggs to the skillet and stir to combine. Serve the cauliflower fried rice with chopped scallions on top.

CHIPOTLE TOFU BURRITO BOWLS

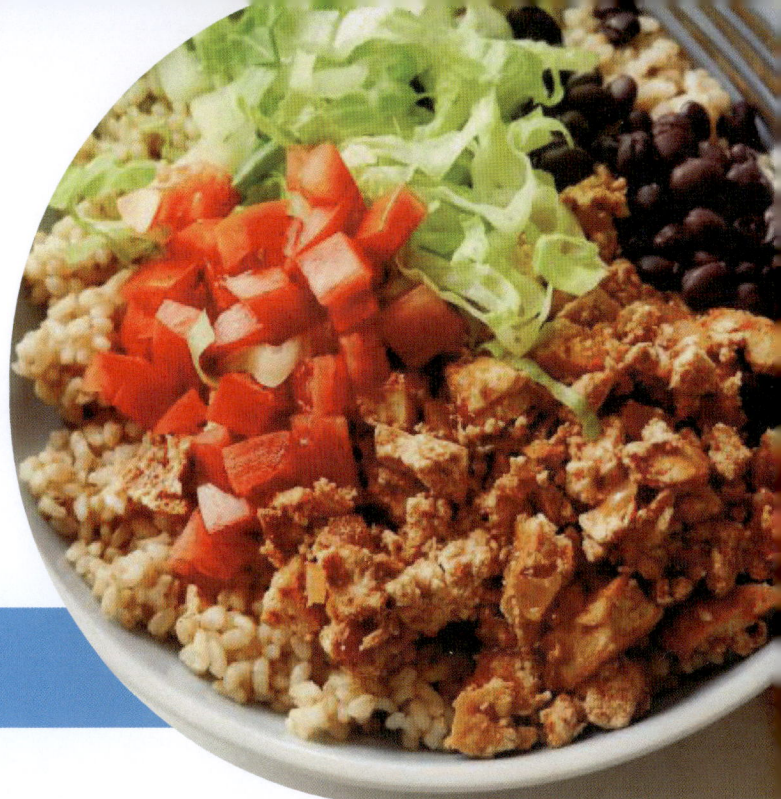

NUTRITION INFORMATION

Calories:	431 Kcal
Protein:	25 g
Carb:	49 g
Fat:	15 g

Prep Time: 30 Minutes	Servings 4

INGREDIENTS

- 1½ blocks of extra firm tofu, cubed
- 1 tablespoon olive oil
- 1 tablespoon chipotle pepper in adobo sauce
- 1 tablespoon honey
- 1 teaspoon ground cumin
- ½ teaspoon garlic powder
- Salt and pepper, to taste
- 1 cup cooked brown rice
- 1 cup canned/cooked black beans, drained and rinsed
- 1 cup corn kernels
- Toppings: diced avocado, sliced jalapeños, chopped cilantro, lime wedges

INSTRUCTIONS

1. Whisk the olive oil with chipotle pepper in adobo sauce, honey, cumin, garlic powder, salt, and pepper in a small bowl. Place the cubed tofu in the marinade and toss to coat evenly. Cover and refrigerate for 30 minutes.
2. Set the air fryer heat to 375°F (190°C). Place the marinated tofu in the air fryer basket and cook for 11-12 minutes; flip after halftime until the tofu is crispy and golden. Mix the cooked brown rice, black beans, and corn kernels in a bowl.
3. Divide the rice and bean mixture among four bowls. Add cooked tofu on top of the rice and bean mixture. Top with diced avocado, sliced jalapeños, chopped cilantro, and a squeeze of lime juice.

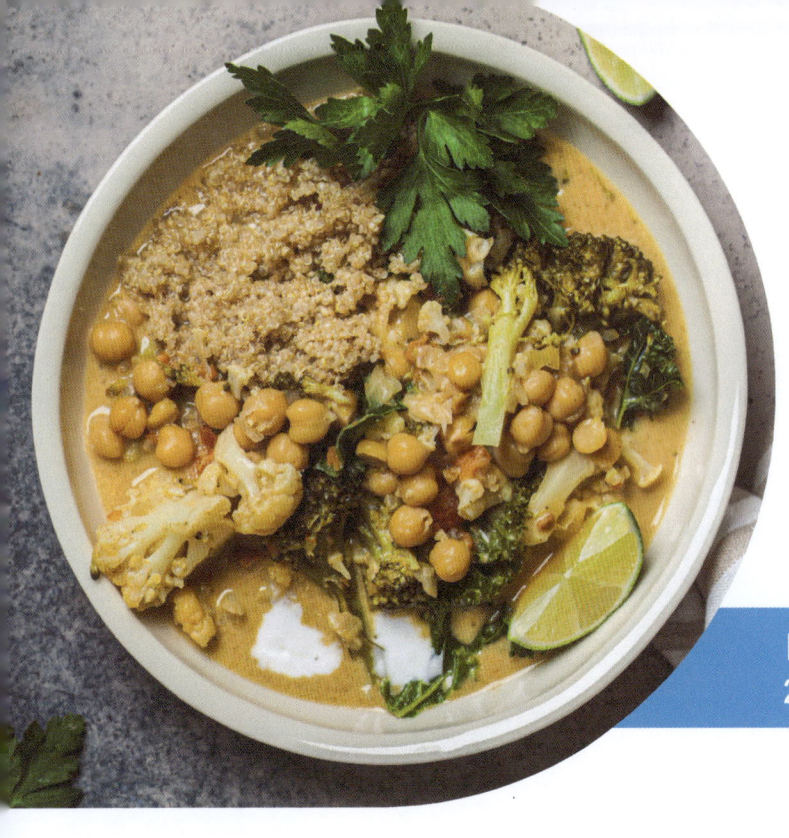

CHICKPEA AND VEGGIE CURRY

NUTRITION INFORMATION

Calories:	361 Kcal
Protein:	29 g
Carb:	23 g
Fat:	17 g

Prep Time: 25 Minutes	Servings 4

INGREDIENTS

- 1 can chickpeas, drained and rinsed
- 1 lb. chicken breast (without skin and bone), chopped like minced
- 1 small onion, chopped
- 2 cloves garlic, minced
- 1 tablespoon olive oil
- 1 tablespoon curry powder
- ½ teaspoon ground cumin
- ½ teaspoon ground turmeric
- Salt and crushed pepper, to taste
- 1 red bell pepper, chopped
- 1 small zucchini, chopped
- ½ cup canned coconut milk
- Chopped cilantro for garnish

INSTRUCTIONS

1. Set the air fryer heat to 400°F (200°C). Mix the chickpeas, onion, garlic, olive oil, curry powder, cumin, turmeric, salt, and pepper in a large bowl. Place the chickpea mixture in the air fryer basket and cook for 8-10 minutes, stirring halfway through, until the chickpeas are lightly browned and crispy.
2. Add the chopped red bell pepper with zucchini and chicken to the basket and cook for 7 minutes, until the veggies are tender. Add canned coconut milk to the air fryer basket and stir to combine.
3. Cook for three minutes until the curry is hot and bubbly. Serve the curry with chopped cilantro on top.

SWEET AND SOUR CHICKEN AND VEGGIES

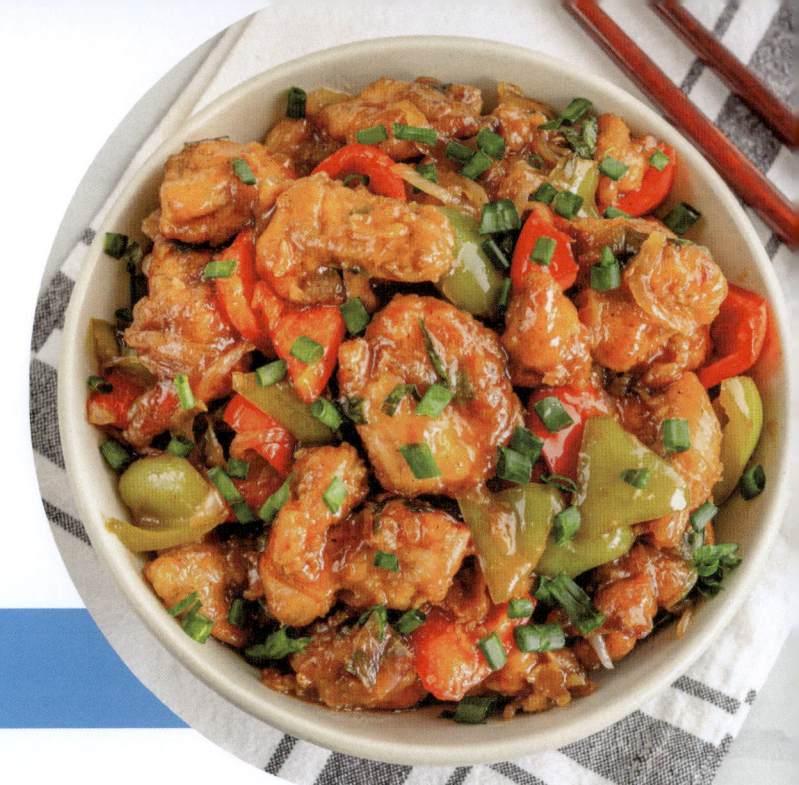

NUTRITION INFORMATION

Calories:	300 Kcal
Protein:	22 g
Carb:	42 g
Fat:	5 g

Prep Time:	Servings
30 Minutes	4

INGREDIENTS

- 1 lb. chicken breasts (without skin & bone), cubed
- 1 tablespoon cornstarch
- Salt and pepper, to taste
- 1 red bell pepper, chopped
- 1 small zucchini, chopped
- 1 small yellow onion, chopped
- ¼ cup pineapple chunks
- ¼ cup ketchup
- ¼ cup apple cider vinegar
- ¼ cup honey
- 2 tablespoons soy sauce
- 1 teaspoon grated ginger
- 1 teaspoon minced garlic
- 1 tablespoon olive oil

INSTRUCTIONS

1. Whisk the cornstarch, salt, and pepper in a small bowl. Add cubed chicken to the cornstarch mixture and toss to coat evenly. Set the air fryer heat to 375°F (190°C). Add chicken into the fryer basket and cook for 11-12 minutes; flip after halftime until the chicken is crispy and cooked.
2. While cooking, whisk the ketchup, apple cider vinegar, honey, soy sauce, ginger, and garlic in a separate bowl. Put the non-stick skillet over medium-high heat, heat the olive oil. Add the chopped red bell pepper, zucchini, and yellow onion and cook for 5-7 minutes, until the veggies are tender.
3. Add pineapple chunks with the sweet and sour sauce and stir to combine. Cook for 3-4 minutes, until the sauce is hot and bubbly. Serve the sweet and sour veggies over the cooked chicken.

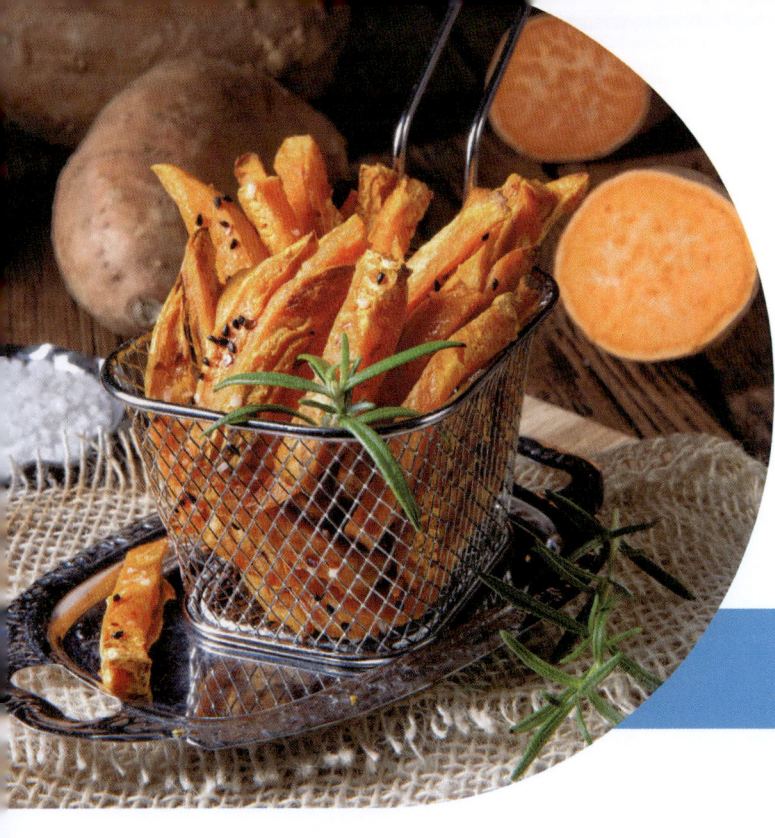

CRISPY SWEET POTATO FRIES

NUTRITION INFORMATION

Calories:	385 Kcal
Protein:	8 g
Carb:	27 g
Fat:	7 g

Prep Time: 25 Minutes	Servings 4

INGREDIENTS

- 2 sweet potatoes, peeled, and fries
- 2 tablespoons olive oil
- 1 teaspoon paprika
- ½ teaspoon garlic powder
- ½ teaspoon onion powder
- Salt and pepper, to taste

INSTRUCTIONS

1. In a large bowl, combine sweet potato fries, olive oil, paprika, garlic powder, onion, salt, and crushed pepper. Toss until the fries are evenly coated. Set the air fryer heat to 375°F (190°C).
2. Place the sweet potato fries in one layer in the fryer basket, don't overcrowd them. Cook for 15 minutes, flipping the fries halfway through to ensure even cooking.
3. Remove the fries from the fryer and serve immediately.

GARLIC AND HERB MUSHROOMS

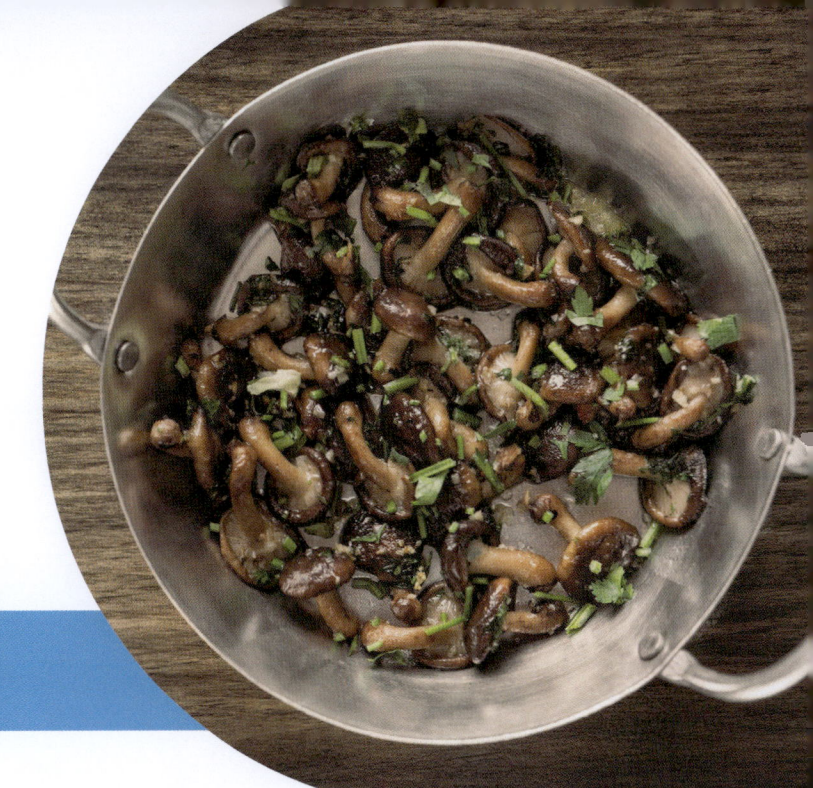

NUTRITION INFORMATION

Calories:	235 Kcal
Protein:	4 g
Carb:	5 g
Fat:	4 g

Prep Time: 22 Minutes	Servings 4

INGREDIENTS

- 1 lb. (450g) white or cremini mushrooms, cleaned and halved
- 2 tablespoons olive oil
- 3 cloves garlic, minced
- 1 teaspoon dried thyme
- 1 teaspoon dried oregano
- Salt and pepper, to taste

INSTRUCTIONS

1. Combine mushrooms, olive oil, garlic, thyme, oregano, salt, and pepper in a large bowl. Toss until the mushrooms are evenly coated.
2. Set the air fryer heat to 350°F (175°C). Put the mushrooms in one layer in the fryer basket. Cook for 09-12 minutes, shaking the basket after halftime to ensure even cooking.
3. Remove the mushrooms from the fryer and serve immediately.

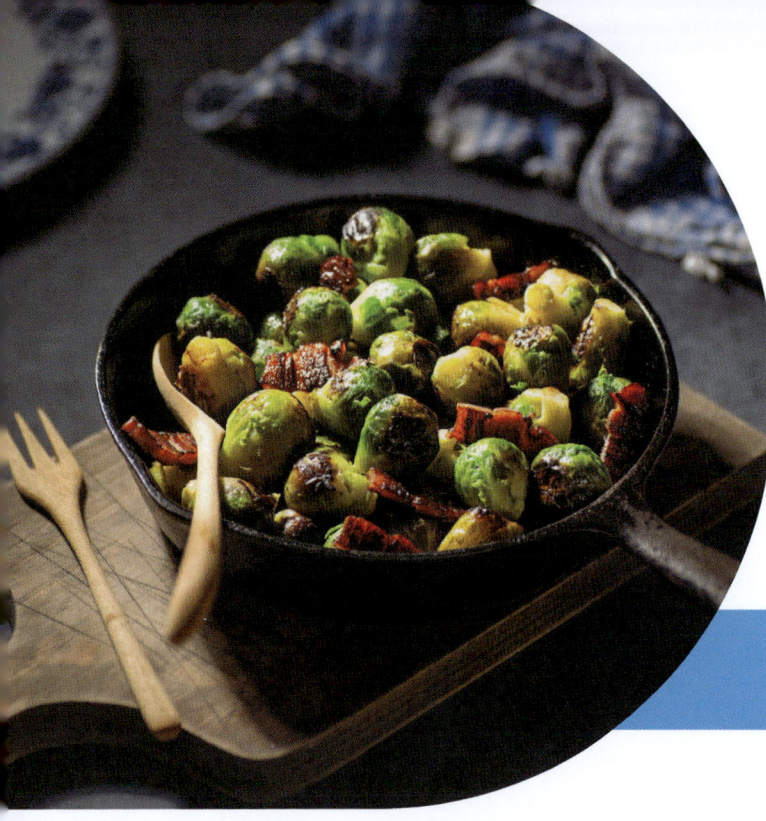

BRUSSELS SPROUTS WITH BALSAMIC GLAZE

NUTRITION INFORMATION

Calories:	244 Kcal
Protein:	9 g
Carb:	24 g
Fat:	9 g

Prep Time: 25 Minutes	Servings 4

INGREDIENTS

- 1 lb. (450g) Brussels sprouts, trimmed and halved
- 2 tablespoons olive oil
- Salt and pepper, to taste
- ¼ cup balsamic vinegar
- 2 tablespoons clear or raw honey or maple syrup (for a vegan option)

INSTRUCTIONS

1. In a bowl, whisk the Brussels sprouts with olive oil, salt, and crushed pepper. Toss until the sprouts are evenly coated. Set the air fryer heat to 375°F (190°C). Place the Brussels sprouts in one layer in the air fryer basket.
2. Cook for 13-15 minutes, shaking the basket thoroughly after halftime to ensure even cooking. While the sprouts cook, prepare the balsamic glaze by combining balsamic vinegar and honey or maple syrup in a small saucepan.
3. Take the mixture to a boil over moderate heat, then decrease the burner heat and simmer for 5-7 minutes. Remove the Brussels sprouts and drizzle with the balsamic glaze. Serve immediately.

SESAME GINGER TOFU

NUTRITION INFORMATION

Calories:	325 Kcal
Protein:	15 g
Carb:	16 g
Fat:	11 g

Prep Time: 22 Minutes	Servings 4

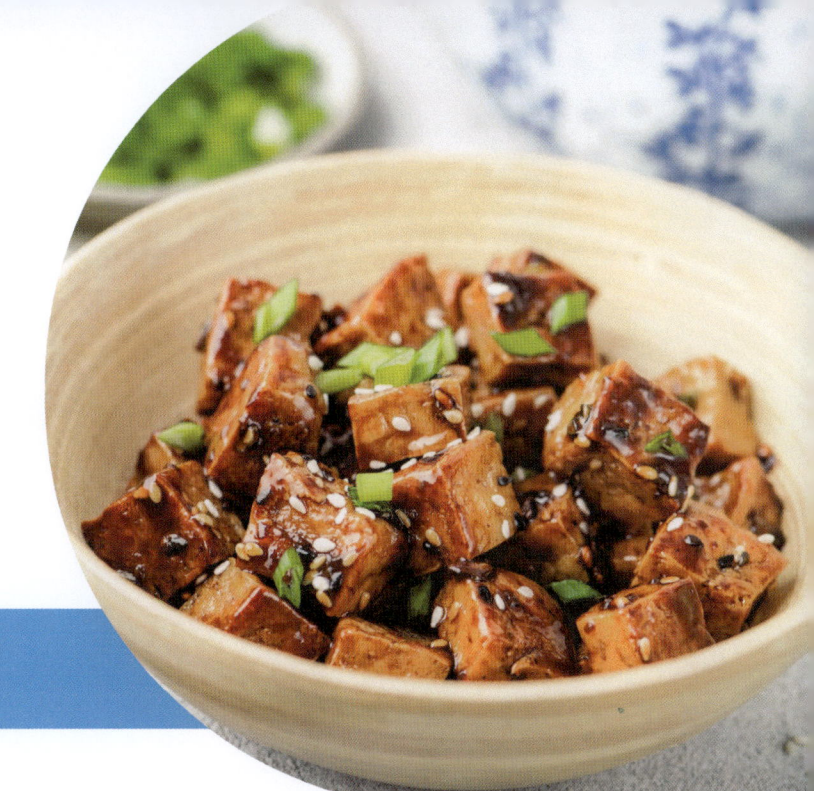

INGREDIENTS

- 1 lb. (450g) extra-firm tofu, pressed and cut into cubes
- 3 tablespoons soy sauce
- 1 tablespoon rice vinegar
- 1 tablespoon maple syrup
- 1 tablespoon sesame oil
- 1 tablespoon minced ginger
- 2 cloves garlic, minced
- 2 tablespoons cornstarch
- 2 tablespoons sesame seeds

INSTRUCTIONS

1. Beat the soy sauce with rice vinegar, maple syrup, sesame oil, ginger, and garlic in a small bowl. Add tofu cubes to the marinade, making sure they are well coated. Allow the tofu to marinate for thirty minutes, stirring occasionally.
2. Set the air fryer heat to 375°F (190°C). Remove the tofu reserving the remaining liquid. Toss the tofu in cornstarch. Place the tofu cubes in one layer in the air fryer basket. Cook for 12 minutes, flipping the tofu halfway through to ensure even cooking.
3. While the tofu cooks, bring the reserved marinade to a boil in a small saucepan. Simmer for three minutes to thicken the sauce. Remove the tofu from the air fryer, drizzle with the thickened sauce, and sprinkle with sesame seeds. Serve immediately.

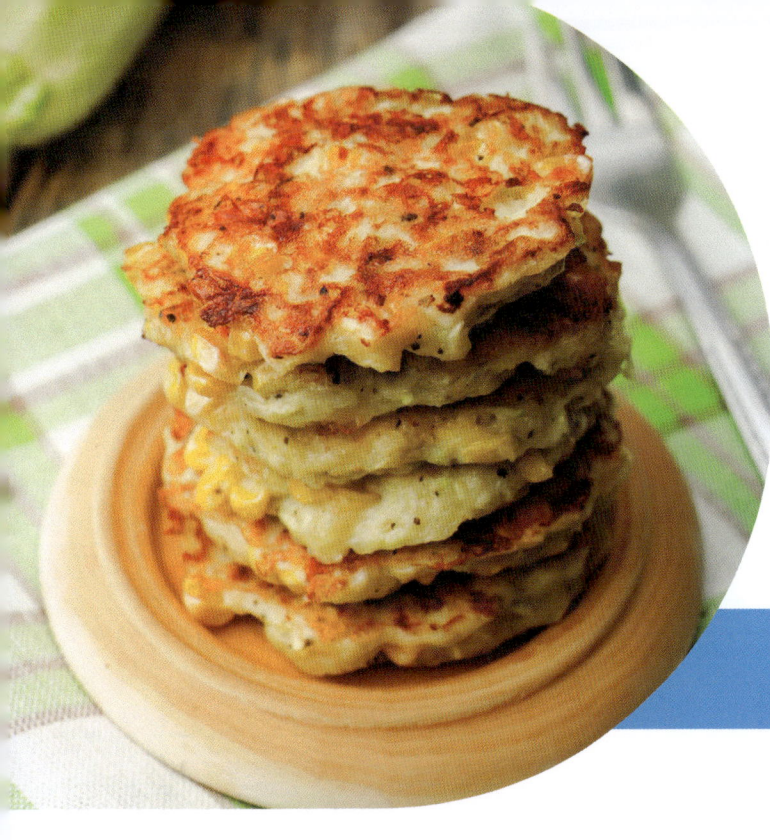

ZUCCHINI AND CORN FRITTERS

NUTRITION INFORMATION

Calories:	250 Kcal
Protein:	6 g
Carb:	26 g
Fat:	5 g

Prep Time: 25 Minutes	Servings 4

INGREDIENTS

- 1 cup grated zucchini, squeezed to remove excess moisture
- 1 cup corn kernels, frozen or fresh (if frozen, then thawed)
- ½ cup all-purpose flour
- ¼ cup grated Parmesan cheese (use vegan cheese for a vegan option)
- ¼ cup chopped scallions
- ½ teaspoon baking powder
- Salt and pepper, to taste

INSTRUCTIONS

1. Combine grated zucchini, corn kernels, flour, Parmesan cheese (or vegan cheese), scallions, baking powder, salt, and pepper in a large bowl. Mix until well combined. Set the air fryer heat to 375°F (190°C). Lightly grease the fryer basket with cooking spray.
2. Shape the zucchini and corn mixture into small patties about 2 inches in diameter. Place the patties in one layer in the fryer basket, ensure not to overcrowd them. Work in batches.
3. Cook for 10 minutes, flipping the fritters halfway to ensure even cooking. Remove the fritters from the air fryer and serve immediately with your favorite dipping sauce.

STUFFED JALAPENO PEPPERS

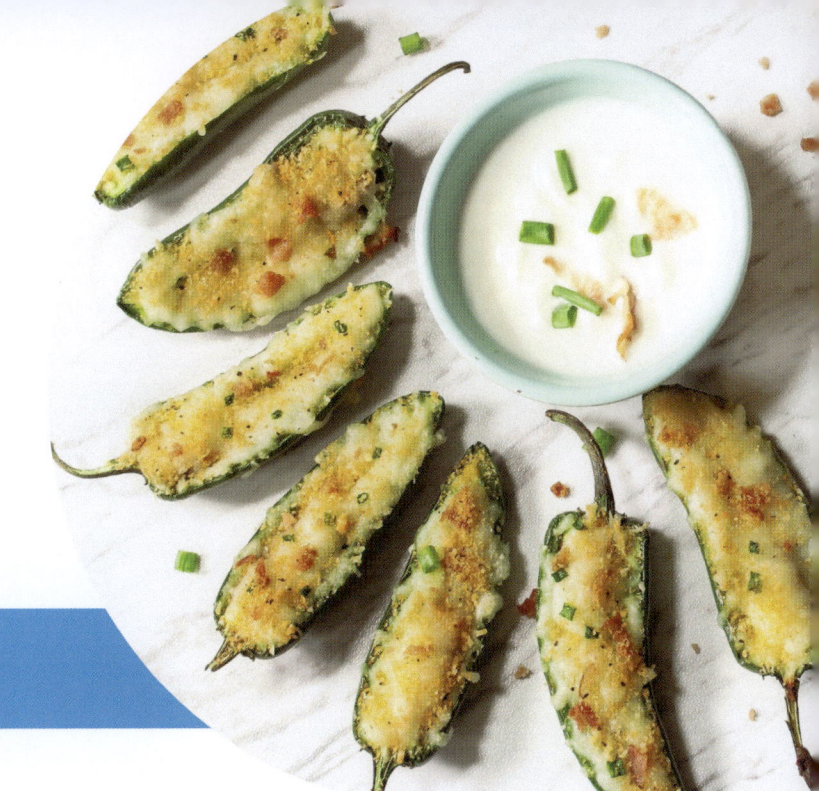

NUTRITION INFORMATION

Calories:	320 Kcal
Protein:	12 g
Carb:	6 g
Fat:	18 g

Prep Time: 35 Minutes	Servings 6

INGREDIENTS

- 12 jalapeno peppers
- 8 oz (225g) cream cheese, softened
- 1 cup shredded cheddar cheese
- ½ teaspoon garlic powder
- ½ teaspoon onion powder
- ½ teaspoon smoked paprika
- ¼ teaspoon ground cumin
- Salt and crushed pepper, to taste
- 6 slices bacon, cut in half crosswise
- Toothpicks for securing bacon

INSTRUCTIONS

1. Set the air fryer heat to 375°F (190°C). Cut the jalapeno peppers lengthwise to seedless using a spoon or a small knife. Beat the softened cream cheese, shredded cheddar cheese, garlic, onion powder, smoked paprika powder, ground cumin, salt, and crushed pepper until well combined.
2. Fill each jalapeno pepper in half with the cream cheese mixture, ensuring it is level with the edges of the pepper. Wrap each stuffed pepper half with ½ bacon slice, securing it with a toothpick if necessary.
3. Place the wrapped jalapeno peppers in one layer in the fryer basket, don't overcrowd them. Work in batches. Cook for 13-15 minutes or until the bacon is crispy and the peppers are tender.
4. Carefully remove the stuffed jalapeno peppers from the air fryer and serve immediately.

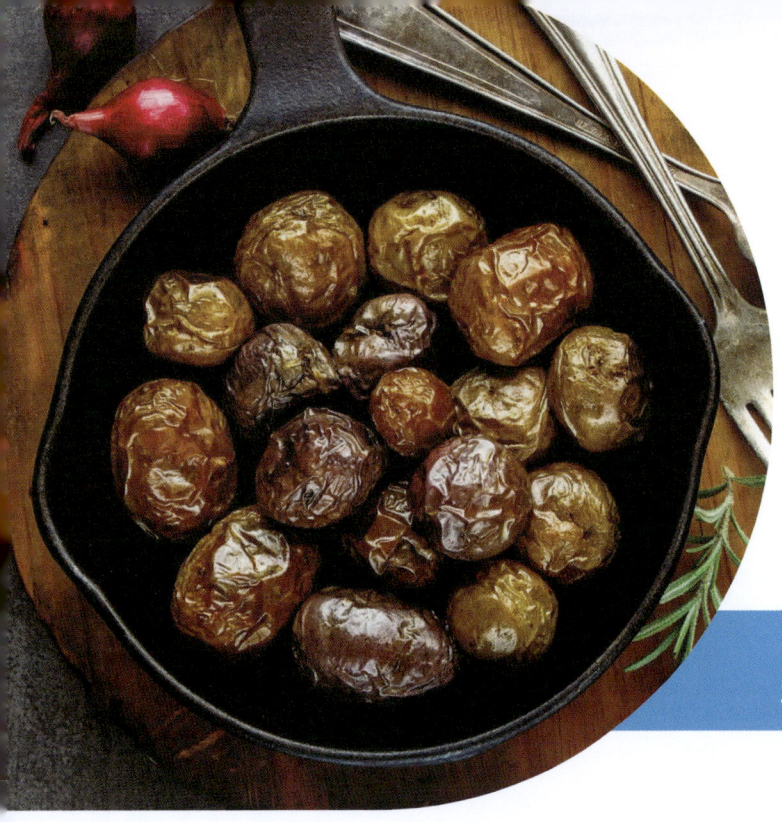

GARLIC ROSEMARY BABY POTATOES

NUTRITION INFORMATION

Calories:	385 Kcal
Protein:	3 g
Carb:	30 g
Fat:	7 g

Prep Time: 30 Minutes	Servings 4

INGREDIENTS

- 1 lb. (450g) baby potatoes, halved
- 2 tablespoons olive oil
- 3 cloves garlic, minced
- 1 tablespoon fresh rosemary, chopped
- Salt and pepper, to taste

INSTRUCTIONS

1. Combine baby potatoes, olive oil, garlic, rosemary, salt, and pepper in a large bowl. Toss until the potatoes are evenly coated. Set the air fryer heat to 400°F (200°C). Place the potatoes in one layer in the air fryer basket.
2. Cook for 17-20 minutes, shaking the basket after halftime to ensure even cooking. Remove the potatoes from the fryer and serve immediately.

AIR FRYER SPICY CHICKPEAS

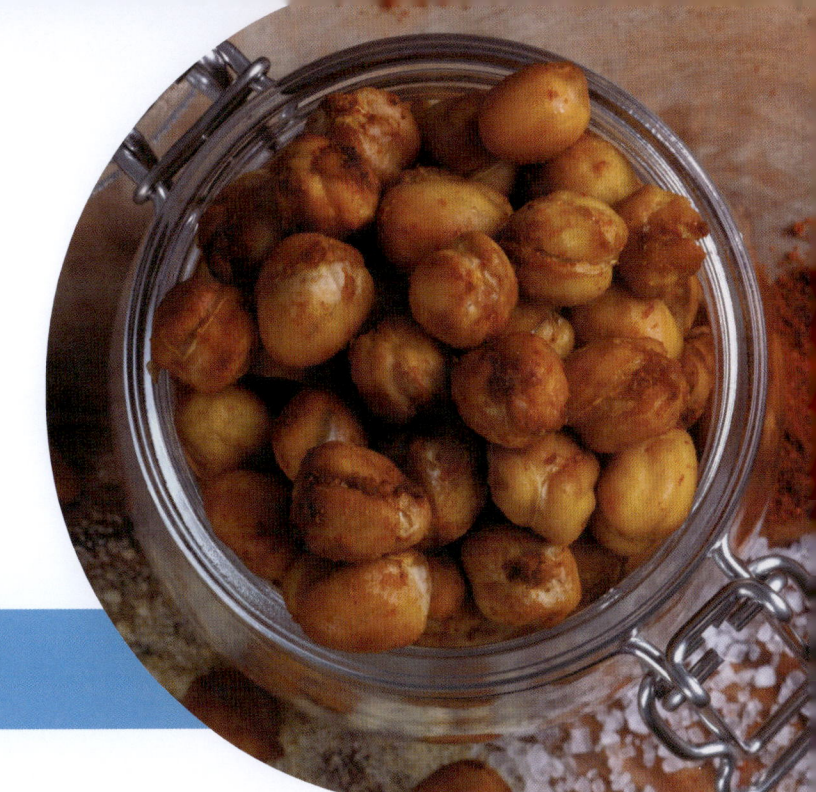

NUTRITION INFORMATION

Calories:	230 Kcal
Protein:	6 g
Carb:	23 g
Fat:	5 g

Prep Time: 20 Minutes	Servings 4

INGREDIENTS

- 2 cups chickpeas (canned), drained and rinsed
- 1 tablespoon olive oil
- ½ teaspoon smoked paprika
- ½ teaspoon ground cumin
- ¼ teaspoon cayenne pepper (adjust to taste)
- Salt, to taste

INSTRUCTIONS

1. Combine chickpeas, olive oil, smoked paprika, cumin, cayenne pepper, and salt in a large bowl. Toss until the chickpeas are evenly coated. Set the air fryer heat to 390°F (200°C). Place the chickpeas in one layer in the air fryer basket.
2. Cook for 13-15 minutes, shaking the basket every 5 minutes to ensure even cooking. Remove the chickpeas from the fryer and serve immediately or let them cool for a crunchy snack.

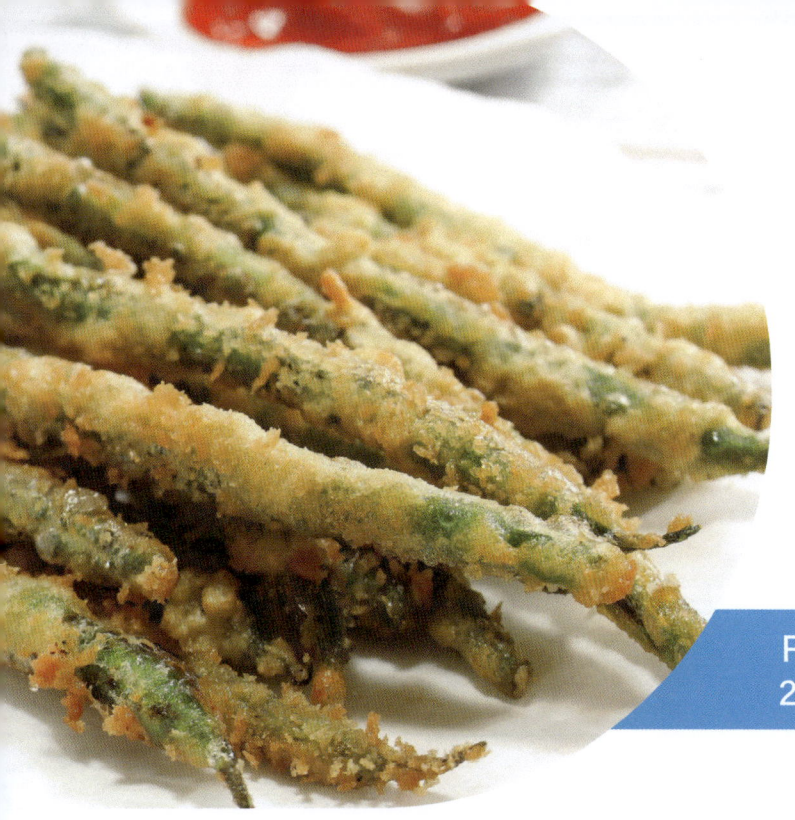

GREEN BEAN FRIES WITH VEGAN AIOLI

NUTRITION INFORMATION

Calories:	385 Kcal
Protein:	5 g
Carb:	45 g
Fat:	14 g

Prep Time: 25 Minutes	Servings 4

INGREDIENTS

- 1 lb. (450g) fresh green beans, trimmed
- ½ cup all-purpose flour
- 2 tablespoons cornstarch
- ½ teaspoon garlic powder
- Salt and pepper, to taste
- ½ cup unsweetened almond milk
- 1 cup panko breadcrumbs
- Cooking spray

Vegan Aioli:
- ½ cup vegan mayonnaise
- 1 tablespoon lemon juice
- 1 clove garlic, minced
- Salt and pepper, to taste

INSTRUCTIONS

1. Combine flour, cornstarch, garlic powder, salt, and pepper in a shallow dish. In the other deep-bottom dish, pour the almond milk. In a third deep-bottom dish, place the panko breadcrumbs. In batches, dip the green beans into the flour mixture, the almond milk, and the breadcrumbs, pressing to coat evenly.
2. Set the air fryer heat to 400°F (200°C) and lightly grease the air fryer basket with cooking spray. Place the coated green beans in one layer in the air fryer basket, ensuring not to overcrowd them. Work in batches.
3. Cook for 10 minutes, flipping the green beans halfway through to ensure even cooking. While the green beans cook, prepare the vegan aioli by mixing vegan mayonnaise, lemon juice, garlic, salt, and crushed pepper in a small bowl.
4. Remove the green beans from the fryer and serve immediately with vegan aioli.

CRISPY BUFFALO CAULIFLOWER

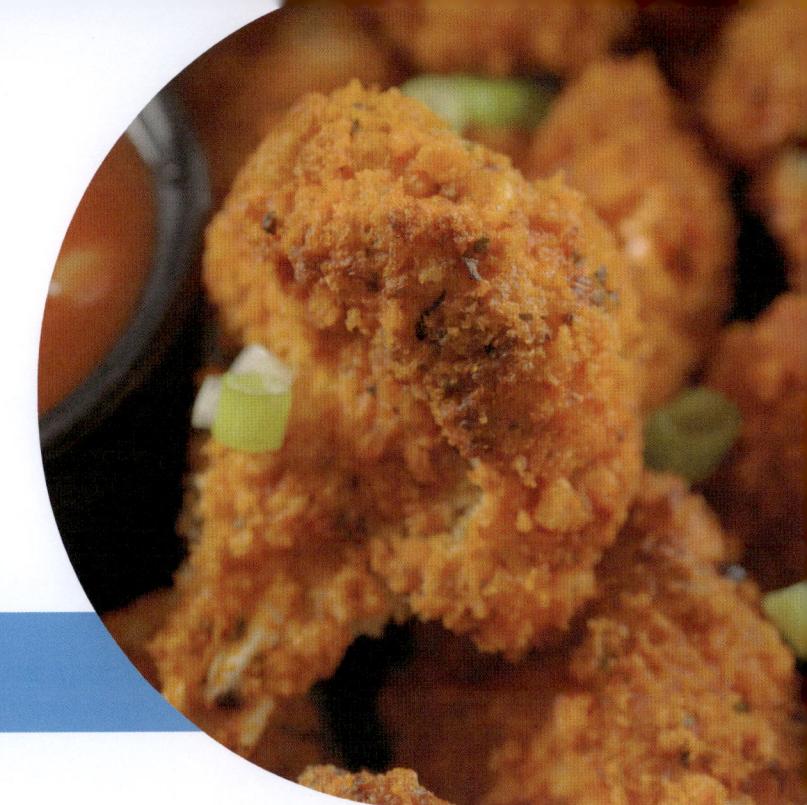

NUTRITION INFORMATION

Calories:	150 Kcal
Protein:	7 g
Carb:	53 g
Fat:	11 g

Prep Time: 35 Minutes	Servings 4

INGREDIENTS

- 1 medium head cauliflower, cut into florets
- 1 cup all-purpose flour
- 1 teaspoon garlic powder
- Salt and pepper, to taste
- 1 cup unsweetened almond/coconut milk
- 1 cup panko breadcrumbs
- ½ cup buffalo hot sauce
- 2 tablespoons vegan butter, melted

INSTRUCTIONS

1. Combine flour with garlic powder, salt, and crushed pepper in the deep-bottom dish. In the other deep-bottom dish, pour the almond milk. In a third deep-bo dish, place the panko breadcrumbs.
2. Working in batches, dip the cauliflower florets first into the flour mixture, then into the almond milk, and finally into the breadcrumbs, pressing to coat evenly. Set the air fryer heat to 375°F (190°C).
3. Place the coated cauliflower in one layer in the air fryer basket, ensuring it does not overcrowd them. Work in batches. Cook for 20 minutes, flipping the cauliflower halfway through to ensure even cooking.
4. In a small saucepan, combine buffalo hot sauce and vegan butter. Heat over low flame until the butter is melted, then whisk to combine. Remove the cauliflower from the air fryer, toss with the buffalo sauce, and serve immediately.

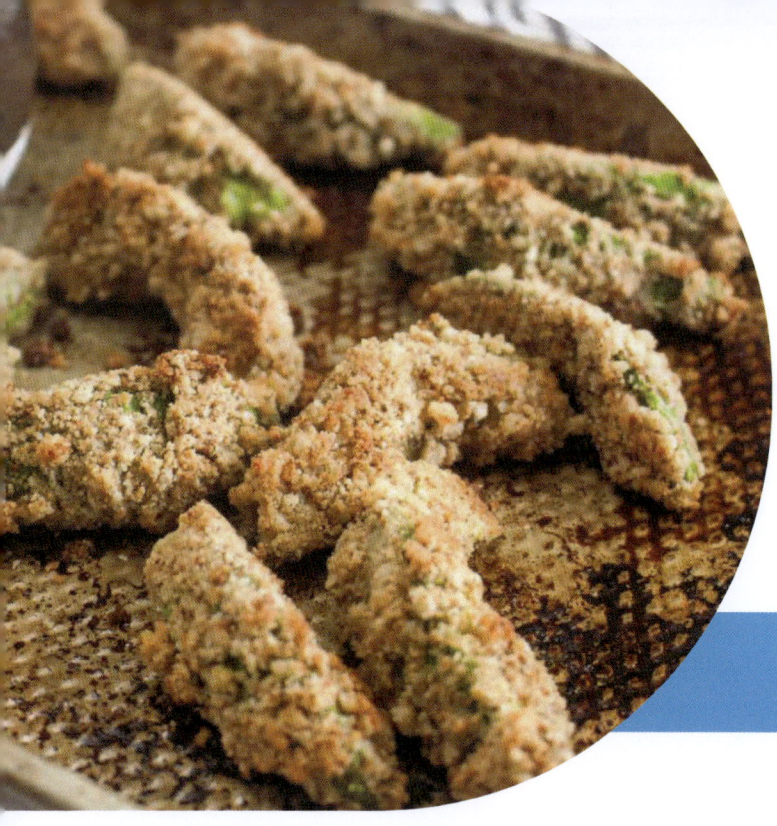

AVOCADO FRIES WITH CILANTRO LIME DIPPING SAUCE

NUTRITION INFORMATION

Calories:	135 Kcal
Protein:	5 g
Carb:	35 g
Fat:	16 g

Prep Time:	Servings
25 Minutes	4

INGREDIENTS

- 2 ripe, firm avocados, peeled, pitted, and sliced
- ½ cup all-purpose flour
- Salt and pepper, to taste
- 1 cup panko breadcrumbs
- ½ cup milk
- Cooking spray

Cilantro Lime Dipping Sauce:
- ½ cup sour cream
- ¼ cup chopped cilantro
- 1 tablespoon lime juice
- Salt and pepper, to taste

INSTRUCTIONS

1. In the deep-bottom dish, combine flour, salt, and crushed pepper. In another shallow dish, pour the milk. In a third deep-bottom dish, place the panko breadcrumbs. Work in batches; dip the avocado wedges first in the flour mix, then into the milk, and finally into the breadcrumbs, pressing to coat evenly.
2. Set the air fryer heat to 400°F (200°C) and lightly grease the air fryer basket with cooking spray. Place the coated avocado wedges in one layer in the fryer basket, don't overcrowd them. Work in batches.
3. Cook for 10 minutes, flipping the avocado wedges halfway through to ensure even cooking. While the avocado fries cook, prepare the cilantro lime dipping sauce by mixing sour cream (vegan sour cream), cilantro, lime juice, salt, and crushed pepper in a small bowl.
4. Remove the avocado fries from the air fryer and serve immediately with the cilantro lime dipping sauce.

KOREAN BBQ CHICKEN WINGS

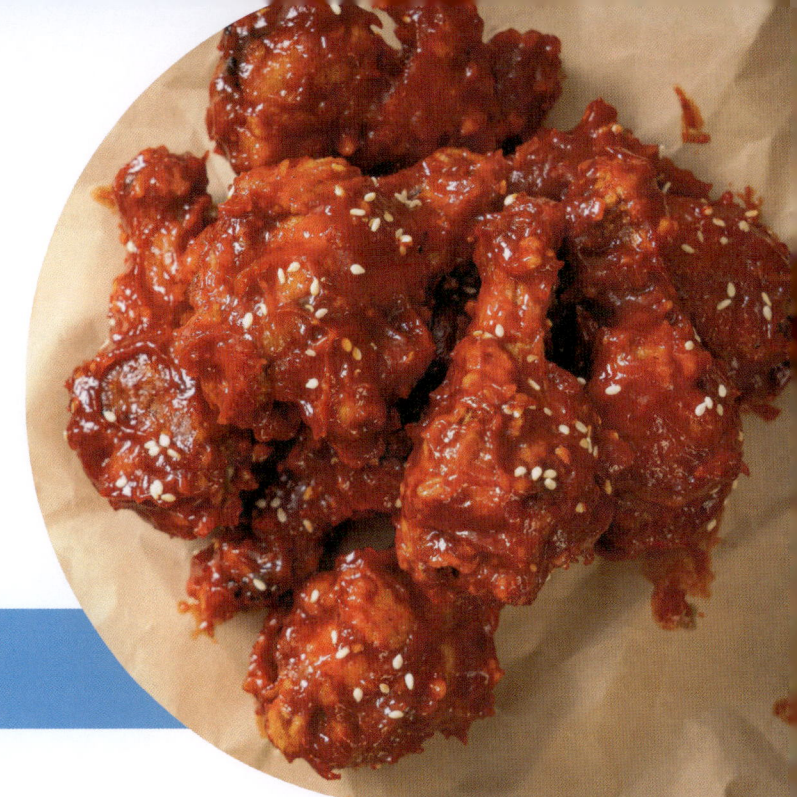

NUTRITION INFORMATION

Calories:	150 Kcal
Protein:	22 g
Carb:	25 g
Fat:	12 g

Prep Time: 35 Minutes	Servings 4

INGREDIENTS

- 2 lb. (900g) chicken wings, tips removed
- ½ cup soy sauce
- ¼ cup honey
- ¼ cup gochujang (Korean red pepper paste)
- 2 tablespoons rice vinegar
- 2 cloves garlic, minced
- 1 tablespoon grated ginger
- 2 green onions, chopped (for garnish)
- Sesame seeds (for garnish)

INSTRUCTIONS

1. Combine soy sauce, honey, gochujang, rice vinegar, garlic, and ginger in a medium bowl. Add chicken wings to the marinade, making sure they are well coated. Marinate the chicken in the refrigerator for thirty minutes or up to 24 hours.
2. Set the air fryer heat to 400°F (200°C). Take out the chicken wings from the marinade, reserving the remaining liquid, and place them in the air fryer basket in one layer. Cook for 25 minutes, flipping the wings halfway through to ensure even cooking.
3. While the chicken cooks, bring the reserved marinade to a boil in a small saucepan. Simmer for four minutes to thicken the sauce. Remove the chicken wings from the fryer, toss with the thickened sauce, and garnish with green onions and sesame seeds. Serve immediately.

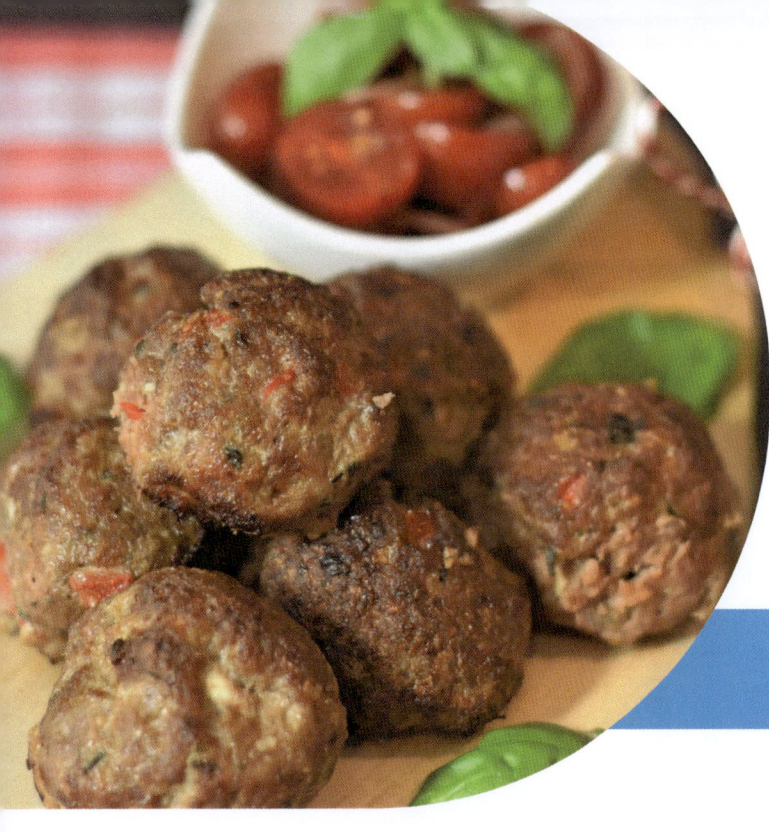

HERBED TURKEY MEATBALLS

NUTRITION INFORMATION

Calories:	385 Kcal
Protein:	25 g
Carb:	8 g
Fat:	12 g

Prep Time: 30 Minutes	Servings 4

INGREDIENTS

- 1 lb. (450g) ground turkey
- ¼ cup breadcrumbs
- ¼ cup grated Parmesan cheese
- ¼ cup chopped fresh parsley
- ¼ cup chopped fresh basil
- ¼ cup chopped fresh chives
- 1 egg, beaten
- 2 cloves garlic, minced
- Salt and pepper, to taste

INSTRUCTIONS

1. Combine ground turkey, breadcrumbs, Parmesan cheese, parsley, basil, chives, egg, garlic, salt, and pepper in a large bowl. Mix until well combined. Shape the mixture into 1.5-inch diameter meatballs.
2. Set the air fryer heat to 375°F (190°C). Put the meatballs in one layer in the fryer basket, don't overcrowd them. Work in batches. Cook for 13-15 minutes until the meatballs are done completely.
3. Remove the meatballs from the fryer and serve immediately.

LEMON HERB CHICKEN DRUMETTES

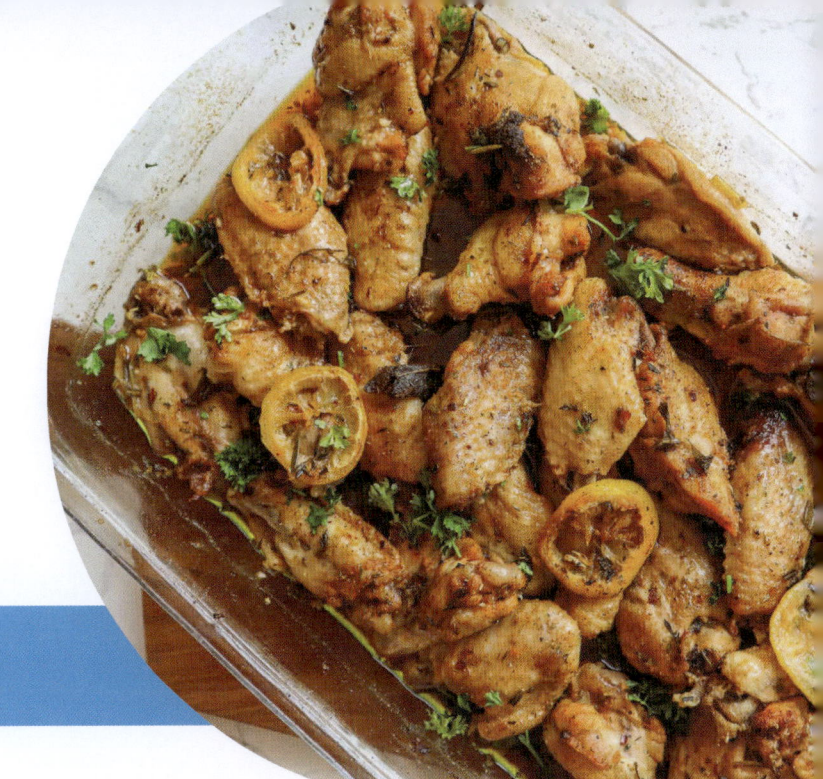

NUTRITION INFORMATION

Calories:	235 Kcal
Protein:	27 g
Carb:	2 g
Fat:	20 g

Prep Time: 35 Minutes	Servings 4

INGREDIENTS

- 2 lb. (900g) chicken drumettes
- ¼ cup olive oil
- ¼ cup lemon juice
- 1 tablespoon lemon zest
- 2 cloves garlic, minced
- 1 tablespoon chopped fresh rosemary
- 1 tablespoon chopped fresh thyme
- Salt and pepper, to taste

INSTRUCTIONS

1. Add olive oil with lemon juice, zest, minced garlic, rosemary, thyme, salt, and crushed pepper in a bowl. Add chicken drumettes to the marinade, making sure they are well coated. Marinate the chicken in the refrigerator for thirty minutes or up to 4 hours.
2. Set the air fryer heat to 400°F (200°C). Remove the chicken drumettes from the marinade, shake off any excess, then put them in the air fryer basket in one layer. Cook for 25 minutes, flipping the drumettes halfway to ensure even cooking.
3. Remove the chicken drumettes from the air fryer and serve immediately.

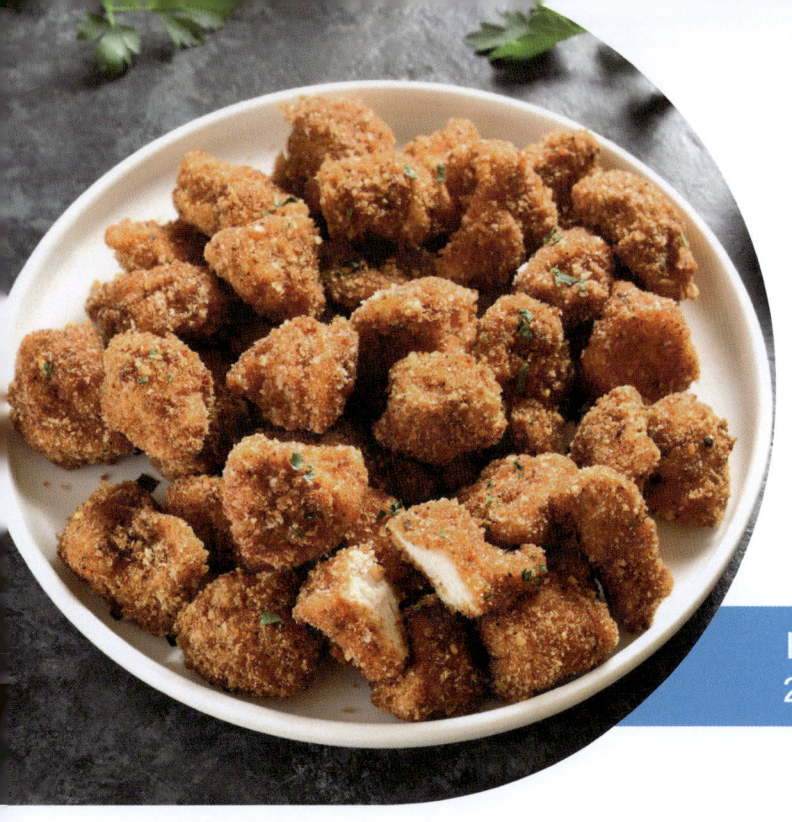

CRISPY FRIED CHICKEN LIVERS

NUTRITION INFORMATION

Calories:	320 Kcal
Protein:	20 g
Carb:	25 g
Fat:	8 g

Prep Time: 22 Minutes	Servings 4

INGREDIENTS

- 1 lb. (450g) chicken livers, trimmed and patted dry
- 1 cup buttermilk
- 1 cup all-purpose flour
- 1 teaspoon paprika
- 1 teaspoon garlic powder
- 1 teaspoon onion powder
- Salt and pepper, to taste
- Cooking spray

INSTRUCTIONS

1. Place chicken livers in a bowl, pour buttermilk over them, and ensure they are fully coated. Allow the livers to soak for at least 30 minutes. Whisk the flour with paprika, garlic powder, onion powder, salt, and crushed pepper in a shallow dish.
2. Remove the chicken livers from the buttermilk, allowing any excess to drip off. Dredge the livers in the flour mixture, ensuring they are evenly coated. Set the air fryer heat to 400°F (200°C) and lightly grease the air fryer basket with cooking spray.
3. Place the coated chicken livers in one layer in the air fryer basket, ensuring not to overcrowd them. Work in batches. Cook for 12 minutes, flipping the chicken livers halfway through to ensure even cooking.
4. Remove the chicken livers from the air fryer and serve immediately.

BACON-WRAPPED JALAPEÑO POPPERS

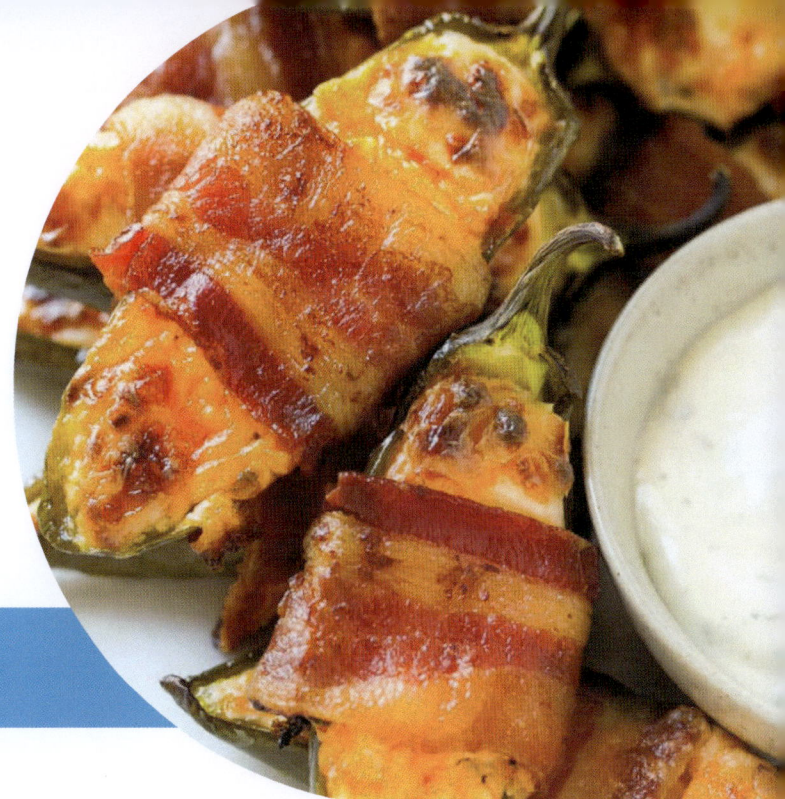

NUTRITION INFORMATION

Calories:	430 Kcal
Protein:	15 g
Carb:	7 g
Fat:	37 g

Prep Time: 25 Minutes	Servings 4

INGREDIENTS

- 8 jalapeños, halved lengthwise and seeds removed
- 8 oz (225g) cream cheese, softened
- 1 cup shredded cheddar cheese
- ½ teaspoon garlic powder
- 16 slices bacon

INSTRUCTIONS

1. Beat the cream cheese with cheddar and garlic powder in a medium bowl. Mix until well combined. Fill each jalapeño half with the cream cheese mixture. Wrap each jalapeño half with a slice of bacon, securing it with a toothpick if necessary.
2. Set the air fryer heat to 375°F (190°C). Place the bacon-wrapped jalapeños in one layer in the fryer basket, don't overcrowd them, and work in batches. Cook for 9-10 minutes or until the bacon is crispy and the jalapeños are tender.
3. Remove the jalapeño peppers from the air fryer and serve immediately.

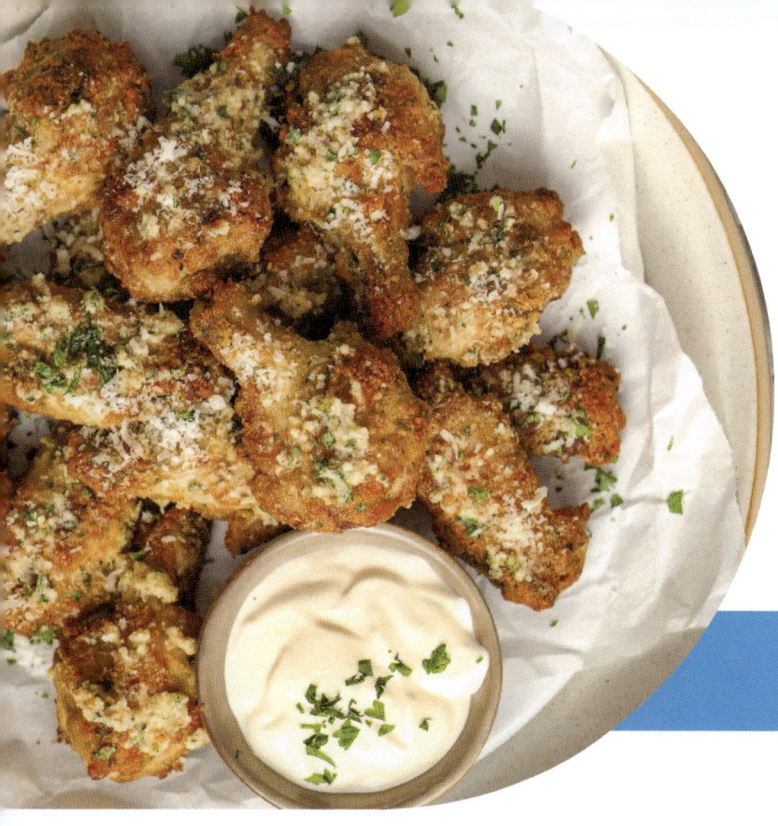

GARLIC PARMESAN CHICKEN WINGS

NUTRITION INFORMATION

Calories:	430 Kcal
Protein:	28 g
Carb:	2 g
Fat:	37 g

Prep Time:	Servings
35 Minutes	4

INGREDIENTS

- 2 lb. (900g) chicken wings, tips removed and separated
- 1 tablespoon olive oil
- Salt and crushed pepper, to taste
- ½ cup grated Parmesan cheese
- 2 cloves garlic, minced
- ¼ cup chopped fresh parsley

INSTRUCTIONS

1. Toss chicken wings with oil, salt, and crushed pepper until well coated. Set the air fryer heat to 400°F (200°C). Place the chicken wings in one layer in the air fryer basket, ensuring not to overcrowd them and work in batches.
2. Cook for 25 minutes, flipping the wings halfway through to ensure even cooking. In the other bowl, combine Parmesan cheese, garlic, and parsley. Toss the cooked wings in the Parmesan mixture until well coated.
3. Remove the wings from the fryer and serve immediately.

LEMON PEPPER SHRIMP

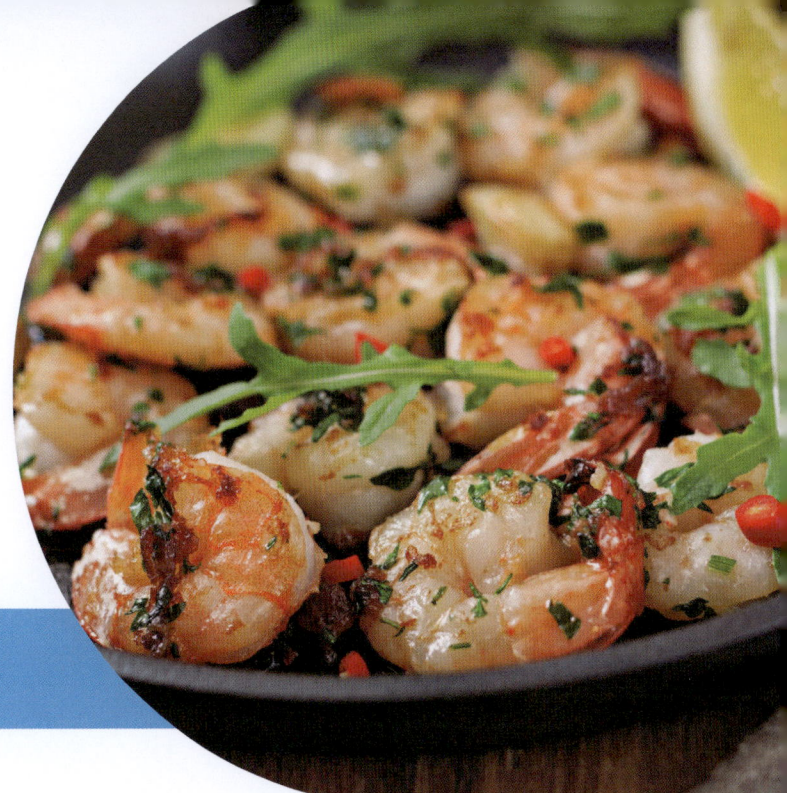

NUTRITION INFORMATION

Calories:	140 Kcal
Protein:	23 g
Carb:	1 g
Fat:	4 g

Prep Time: 16 Minutes	Servings 4

INGREDIENTS

- 1 lb. (450g) shrimp, peeled and deveined
- 1 tablespoon olive oil
- 1 tablespoon lemon juice
- 1 teaspoon lemon zest
- 1 teaspoon freshly ground black pepper
- ½ teaspoon salt
- Chopped fresh parsley for garnish

INSTRUCTIONS

1. Toss shrimp with olive oil, lemon juice, lemon zest, black pepper, and salt until well coated in a large bowl. Set the air fryer heat to 400°F (200°C). Put the shrimp in one layer in the fryer basket, ensuring they do not overcrowd and work in batches.
2. Cook for 6 minutes, flipping the shrimp halfway through to ensure even cooking. Remove the shrimp from the air fryer, garnish with chopped fresh parsley, and serve immediately.

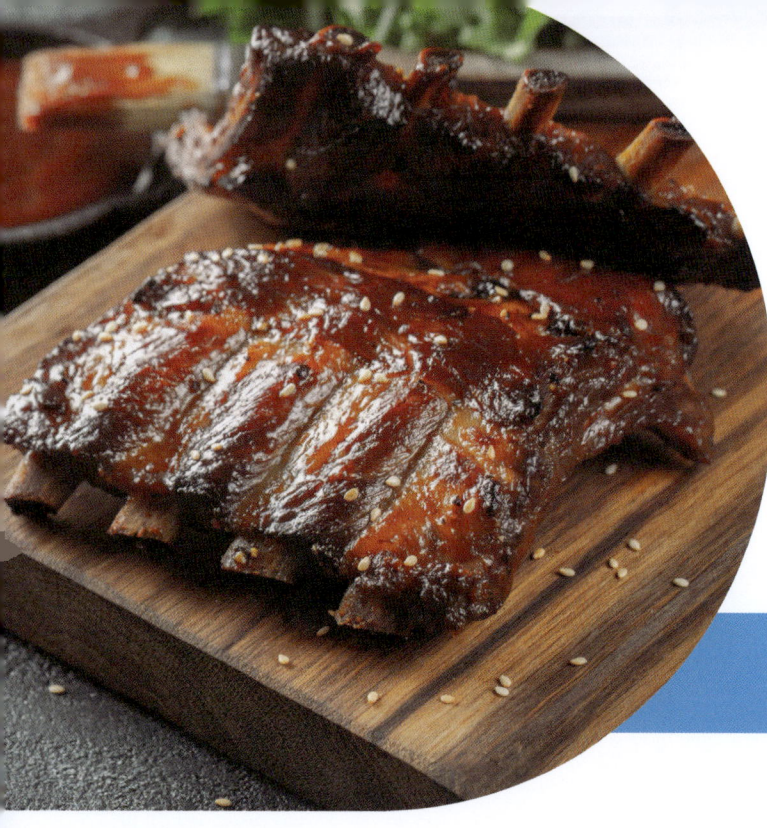

BBQ PORK SPARERIBS

NUTRITION INFORMATION

Calories:	590 Kcal
Protein:	14 g
Carb:	30 g
Fat:	35 g

Prep Time: 40 Minutes	Servings 4

INGREDIENTS

- 2 lb. (900g) pork spareribs, cut into individual ribs
- Salt and pepper, to taste
- 1 cup barbecue sauce

INSTRUCTIONS

1. Season the spareribs with salt and pepper, then put them in the zip-top bag or airtight container. Pour the ½ cup BBQ sauce over the ribs, ensuring they are well coated. Marinate the ribs in the refrigerator for two hours (at least) or up to 24 hours.
2. Set the air fryer heat to 375°F (190°C). Remove the ribs from the zip-lock bag, shaking off any excess, and place them in one layer in the air fryer basket, ensuring not to overcrowd them and work in batches.
3. Cook for 27-30 minutes; flip after halftime to ensure even cooking. In 5 minutes, brush the leftover barbecue sauce over the ribs. Remove the ribs from the fryer and serve immediately.

TERIYAKI CHICKEN SKEWERS

NUTRITION INFORMATION

Calories:	270 Kcal
Protein:	25 g
Carb:	17 g
Fat:	10 g

Prep Time: 30 Minutes	Servings 4

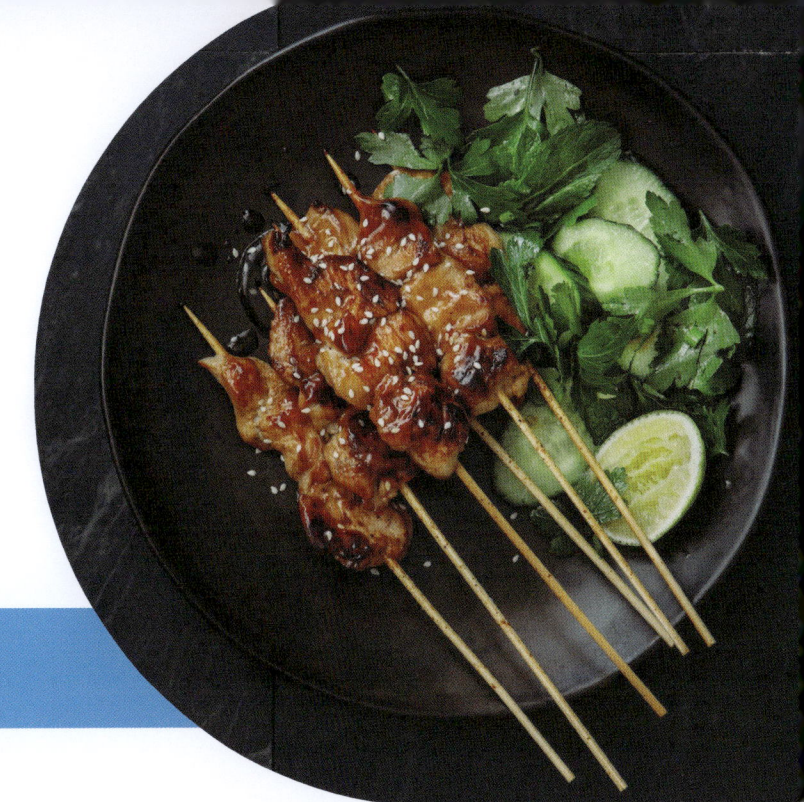

INGREDIENTS

- 1 lb. (450g) chicken thighs (without skin & bone), cut into 1-inch pieces
- ½ cup teriyaki sauce
- 2 bell pepper
- s (red & green), cut into 1-inch pieces
- 1 red onion, cut into 1-inch pieces
- 8 wooden skewers, first soaked them for 30 minutes

INSTRUCTIONS

1. Combine chicken pieces and teriyaki sauce in a large zip-top bag or airtight container. Marinate the chicken in the refrigerator for thirty minutes or up to 4 hours. Set the air fryer heat to 400°F (200°C).
2. Thread the marinated chicken pieces, bell peppers, and red onion onto the soaked wooden skewers, alternating between ingredients. Place the skewers in one layer in the fryer basket, don't overcrowd them, and work in batches.
3. Cook for 12 minutes, flipping the skewers halfway through to ensure even cooking. Remove the skewers from the air fryer and serve immediately.

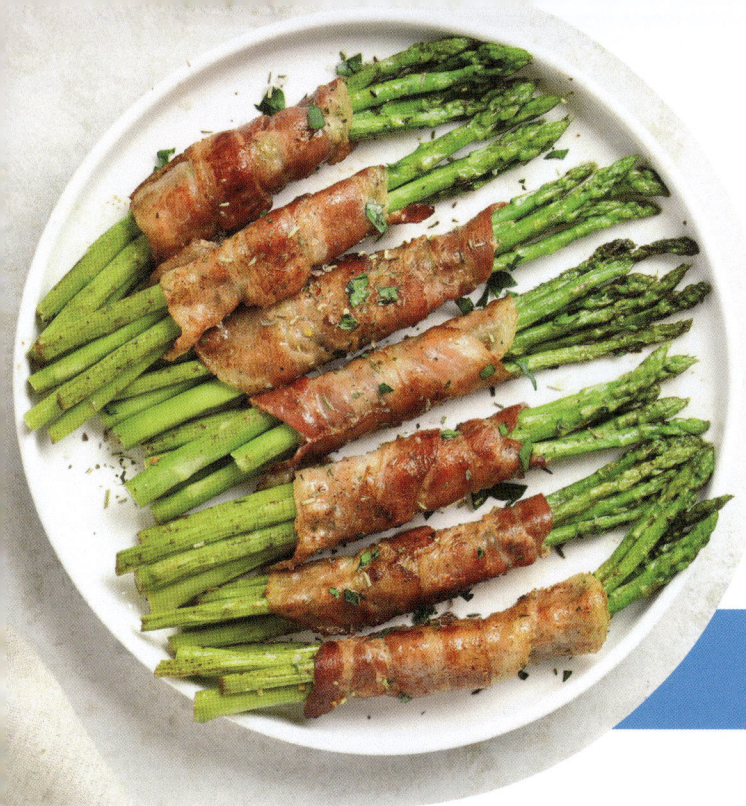

PROSCIUTTO-WRAPPED ASPARAGUS

NUTRITION INFORMATION

Calories:	110 Kcal
Protein:	10 g
Carb:	3 g
Fat:	6 g

Prep Time:	Servings
17 Minutes	4

INGREDIENTS

- 16 asparagus spears, trimmed
- 16 thin slices prosciutto
- Olive oil spray

INSTRUCTIONS

1. Wrap one/two asparagus spears with a slice of prosciutto. Set the air fryer heat to 400°F (200°C). Place the prosciutto-wrapped asparagus spears in one layer in the fryer basket, don't overcrowd them, and work in batches.
2. Lightly spray the wrapped asparagus with olive oil. Cook for 7 minutes or until the prosciutto is crispy and the asparagus is tender. Remove the asparagus from the fryer basket and serve immediately.

PARMESAN CRUSTED CHICKEN TENDERS

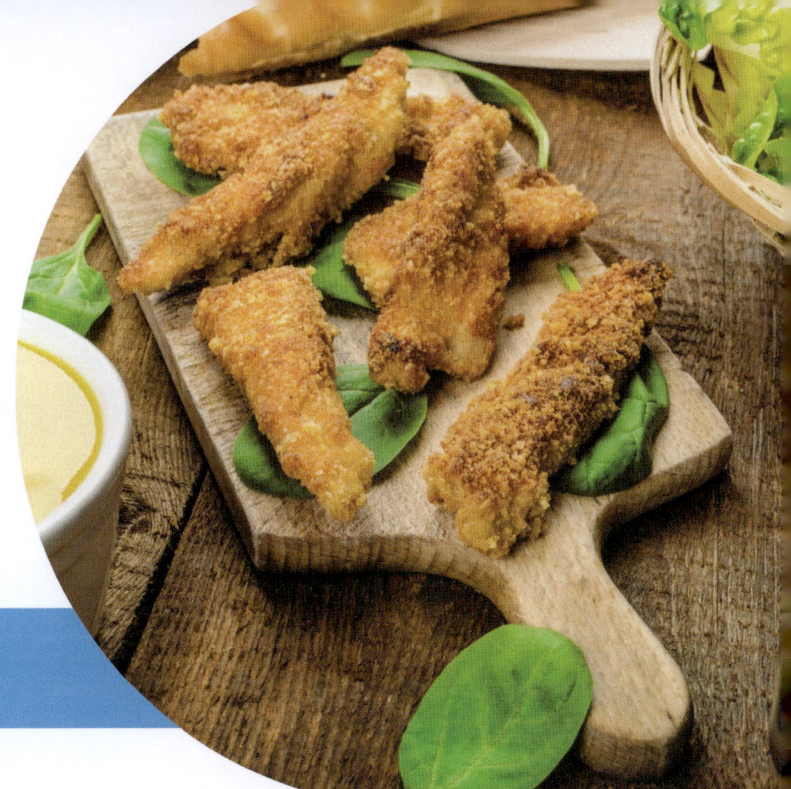

NUTRITION INFORMATION

Calories:	410 Kcal
Protein:	33 g
Carb:	32 g
Fat:	15 g

Prep Time: 27 Minutes	Servings 4

INGREDIENTS

- 1 lb. (450g) chicken tenders
- ½ cup all-purpose flour
- ½ teaspoon salt
- ¼ teaspoon black pepper
- 2 eggs, beaten
- 1 cup panko breadcrumbs
- ½ cup grated Parmesan cheese
- ½ teaspoon garlic powder
- ½ teaspoon dried basil

INSTRUCTIONS

1. In the deep-bottom dish, combine flour, salt, and pepper. In another dish, place the beaten eggs. Combine the panko breadcrumbs with Parmesan cheese, garlic powder, and dried basil in a third dish.
2. Dredge each chicken tenderly in three mixtures, the first flour mixture, the second egg, and then the breadcrumb mixture, pressing to help them adhere. Set the air fryer heat to 400°F (200°C).
3. Put the bread-crusted chicken tenders in one layer in the air fryer basket, ensuring not to overcrowd them and work in batches. Cook for 12 minutes, flipping the tenders halfway to ensure even cooking.
4. Remove the chicken from the fryer and serve immediately.

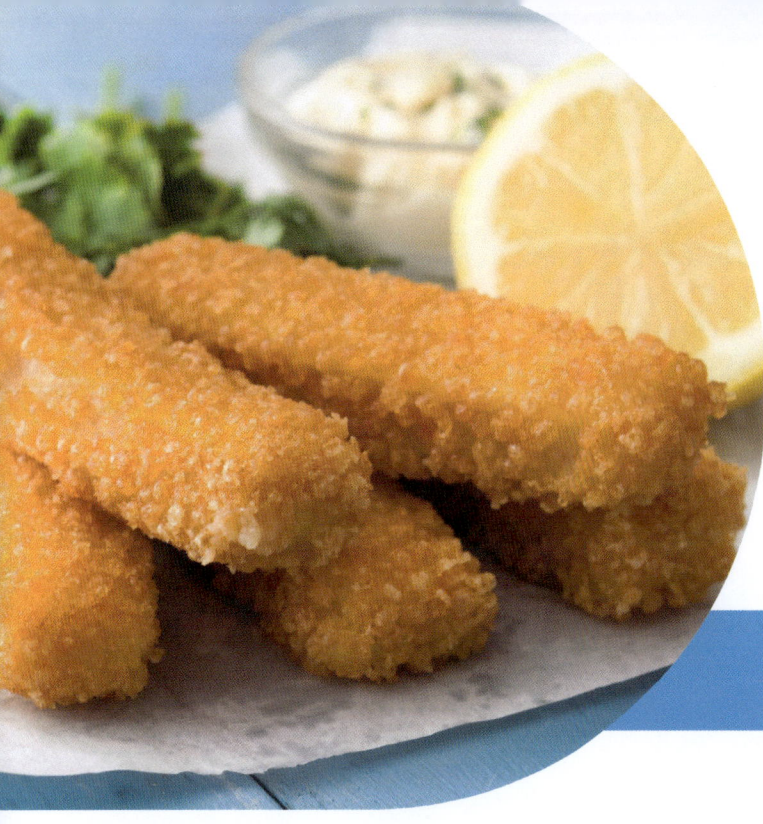

PANKO-CRUSTED FISH STICKS

NUTRITION INFORMATION

Calories:	300 Kcal
Protein:	27 g
Carb:	30 g
Fat:	7 g

Prep Time: 27 Minutes	Servings 4

INGREDIENTS

- 1 lb. (450g) white fish fillets (such as cod or haddock) cut into strips
- ½ cup all-purpose flour
- ½ teaspoon salt
- ¼ teaspoon black pepper
- 2 eggs, beaten
- 1 cup panko breadcrumbs
- ½ teaspoon paprika
- ½ teaspoon dried parsley
- Cooking spray

INSTRUCTIONS

1. In the deep-bottom dish, combine flour, salt, and pepper. In another dish, place the beaten eggs. Combine panko breadcrumbs, paprika, and dried parsley in a third dish. Put the fish strips through three rounds of dredging: flour, egg, and breadcrumb mixture.
2. Press the breadcrumbs onto the fish to help them stick. Set the air fryer heat to 400°F (200°C) and lightly grease the air fryer basket with cooking spray. Place the breaded fish sticks in one layer in the air fryer basket, ensuring not to overcrowd them and work in batches.
3. Lightly spray the fish sticks with cooking spray. Cook for 12 minutes, flipping the fish sticks halfway through to ensure even cooking. Remove the fish sticks from the fryer and serve immediately.

CRISPY ONION RINGS

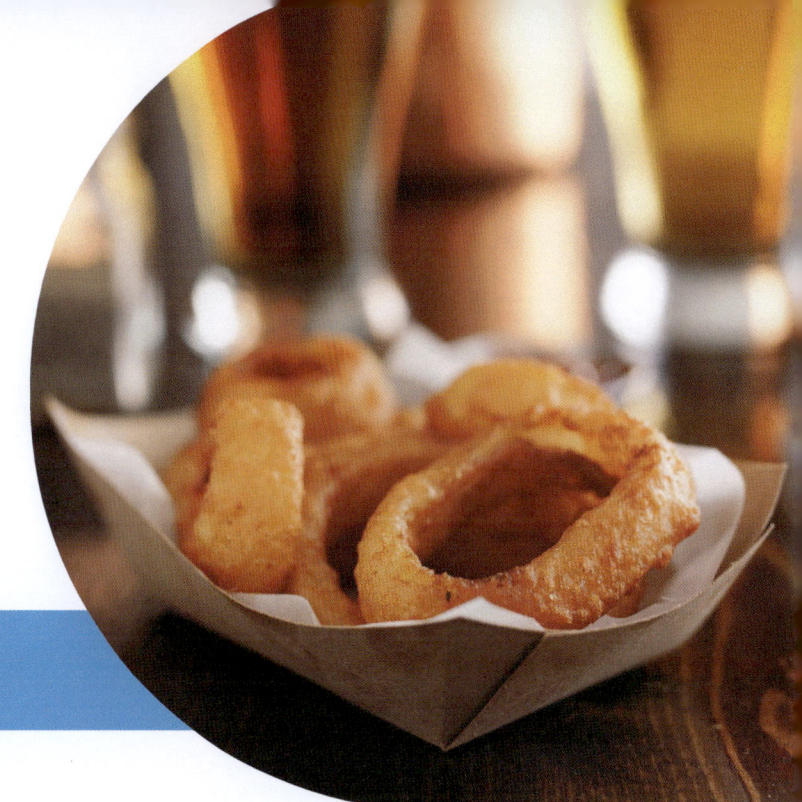

NUTRITION INFORMATION

Calories:	250 Kcal
Protein:	9 g
Carb:	40 g
Fat:	5 g

Prep Time: 25 Minutes	Servings 4

INGREDIENTS

- 1 large onion, cut into half-inch thick slices and separated into rings
- ½ cup all-purpose flour
- ½ teaspoon salt
- ¼ teaspoon black pepper
- 2 eggs, beaten
- 1 cup panko breadcrumbs
- ½ teaspoon paprika
- ½ teaspoon garlic powder
- Cooking spray

INSTRUCTIONS

1. In the deep-bottom dish, combine flour, salt, and pepper. In another dish, place the beaten eggs. Combine panko breadcrumbs, paprika, and garlic powder in a third dish. Dredge each onion ring with three mixtures: flour mixture, egg, and breadcrumb mixture, pressing the breadcrumbs onto the onion to help them adhere.
2. Set the air fryer heat to 400°F (200°C) and lightly grease the air fryer basket with cooking spray. Place the breaded onion rings in one layer in the fryer basket, don't overcrowd them, and work in batches. Lightly spray the onion rings with cooking spray.
3. Cook for 10 minutes, flipping the onion rings halfway through to ensure even cooking. Remove the onion rings from the fryer basket and serve immediately.

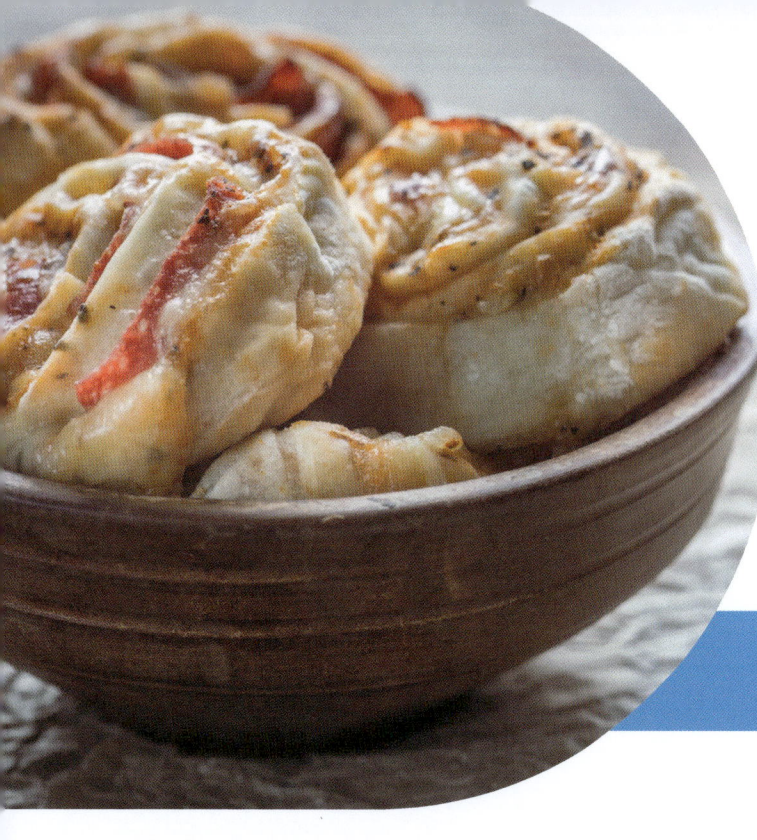

MINI PEPPERONI PIZZA ROLLS

NUTRITION INFORMATION

Calories:	360 Kcal
Protein:	12 g
Carb:	30 g
Fat:	22 g

Prep Time: 28 Minutes	Servings 4

INGREDIENTS

- 1 can (8 oz) frozen crescent roll dough
- 1 cup shredded mozzarella cheese
- ½ cup mini pepperoni slices
- ½ cup pizza sauce

INSTRUCTIONS

1. Set the air fryer heat to 375°F (190°C) and lightly grease the air fryer basket with cooking spray. Unroll the frozen crescent roll dough and separate it into triangles. Paste a thin layer of pizza sauce on each triangle, leaving a small border around the edges.
2. Sprinkle mozzarella cheese and mini pepperoni slices over the pizza sauce. Roll up each triangle tightly at the wide end, enclosing the filling. Place the pizza rolls seam-side down in one layer in the air fryer basket, ensuring not to overcrowd them and work in batches.
3. Cook for 7-8 minutes until the rolls are done. Remove the pizza rolls from the fryer basket and serve immediately.

CONCLUSION

Cheers! At the end of Protein-Packed Air Fryer Meals, the cookbook is filled with 75 delicious and nutritious high-protein meals that can be easily prepared in an air-fryer. We hope this cookbook has inspired you to try new recipes and experiment with air-frying. Whether you're a fitness enthusiast looking to build muscle, a busy professional trying to eat healthy on the go, or simply someone who loves tasty food, there's something in this cookbook for everyone. From juicy burgers to crispy chicken to roasted veggies, there's no shortage of delicious protein-packed options.

We also hope that this cookbook has helped you appreciate the benefits of air frying as a cooking method. Air-frying is healthier and more convenient than traditional frying methods and allows you to create delicious and crispy meals with minimal effort.

At the end of every recipe, we've included nutritional information to help you track your daily protein intake, calories, and other essential nutrients. Healthy food is not always boring, and we hope this cookbook has shown you that healthy food can be both tasty and filling.

Finally, we'd like to thank you for choosing Protein-Packed Air Fryer Meals and for allowing us to be a part of your culinary journey. We hope you've enjoyed using this cookbook as much as we enjoyed creating it. May your air-fryer adventures continue, and may you continue to enjoy healthy, flavorful, and protein-packed meals for years to come!

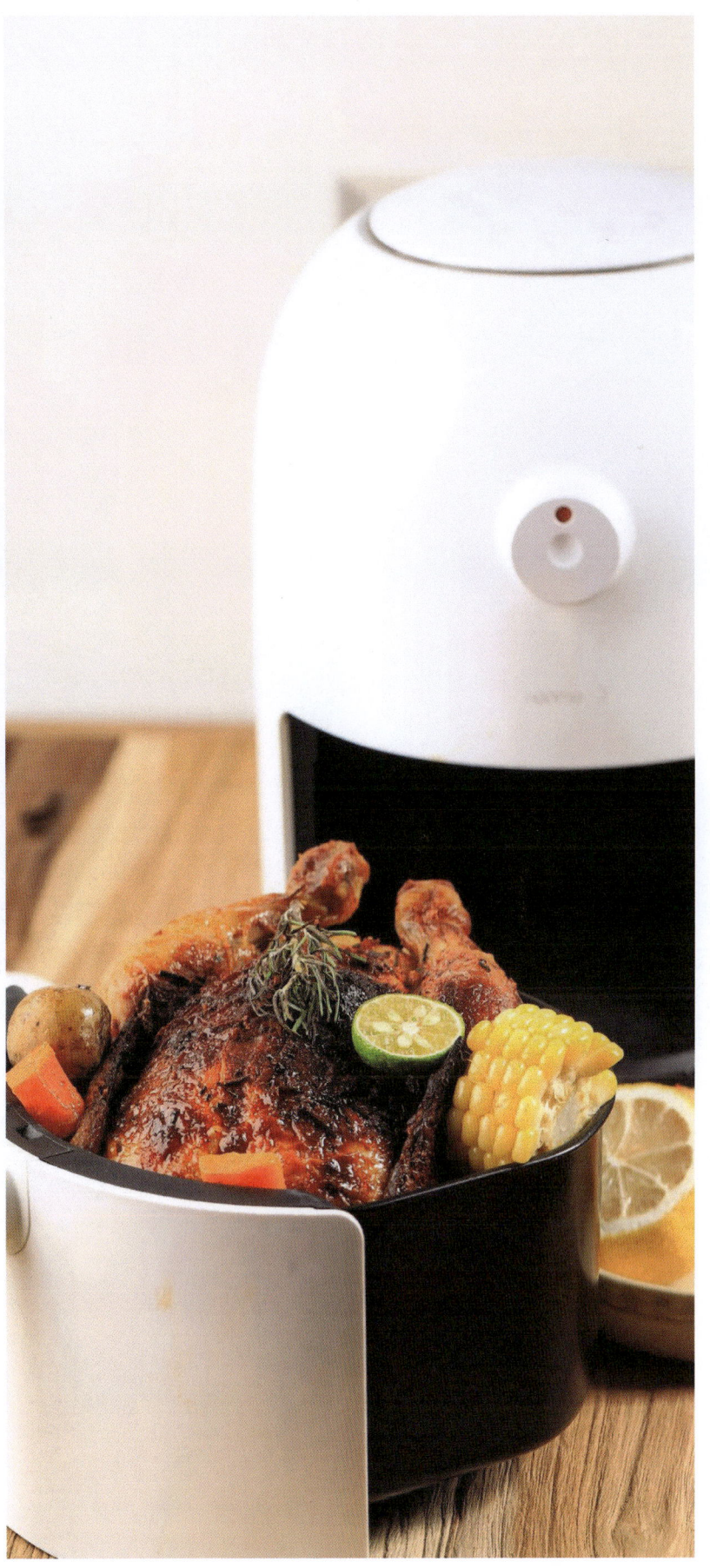

Printed in Great Britain
by Amazon

40884494R00048